D1396135

"Not only is Jon Gabriel genuine in his missio
own weight-loss experience and the skills he acquired in the process, people
respond to his method. If you only read one book on how to focus your mind for
long-term weight loss, make this it."

—Jason Vale (a.k.a. Juice Master), best-selling author, motivational speaker,
and lifestyle coach

"Jon Gabriel's very being resonates with truth and power. What he has done is
available to all of us. I wholeheartedly endorse his latest book on visualization for
weight loss."

—Christiane Northrup, M.D., ob/gyn physician and author of the *New York Times*
bestsellers *Women's Bodies, Women's Wisdom* and *The Wisdom of Menopause*

"Jon Gabriel provides simple, practical ways to use visualization to help reduce
stress and create healthy lifestyle habits that can lead to lasting, sustainable
weight loss."

—Mark Hyman, M.D., author of #1 *New York Times* bestseller
The Blood Sugar Solution 10-Day Detox Diet

"Fast, lasting weight loss goes beyond what you eat or how you exercise. In his
new book, Jon Gabriel provides simple, easy-to-implement strategies to reduce
stress and remove other barriers that create weight loss resistance. If you're doing
everything correctly yet still can't lose weight, visualization could provide the
crucial missing piece of the puzzle. Highly recommended!"

—JJ Virgin, CNS, CHFS, celebrity nutrition and fitness expert and
New York Times best-selling author

"When it comes to weight loss, the mind is as important as the body. I always
say, it's not just about what you're eating—it's also about what's eating you. In
this book, Jon Gabriel teaches simple, practical ways to use your mind to totally
transform your body."

—Kris Carr, *New York Times* best-selling author of *Crazy Sexy Kitchen*

"Jon Gabriel's healing and deep recovery truly come through in these pages.
He shows you how to use your mind to help you lose weight and repair your body
at a cellular level. The hormonal benefits of visualization are well documented,
and I recommend them highly."

—Sara Gottfried M.D., *New York Times* best-selling author of *The Hormone Cure*

"*Visualization for Weight Loss* is a game changer. If using your mind to lose weight
seems too simple to be true, then you haven't yet experienced the power of your
brain's neural pathways on your *body's* biochemistry. The Gabriel Method is easy,
very do-able, and it works!"

—Donna Gates, founder of Body Ecology and author of *The Body Ecology Diet*
and *The Body Ecology Guide to Growing Younger*

"If you're heartbroken from failed weight-loss attempts and tired of feeling at war with your body, it's time for this book. Filled with eye-opening research, powerful tools, and practical tips, it will guide you to harness the power of your mind and body to achieve the weight loss (and life) you want!"

—Jessica Ortner, *New York Times* best-selling author of *The Tapping Solution for Weight Loss and Body Confidence*

"Weight loss is about so much more than calorie math. There are myriad biochemical, mental, and emotional factors that go into the equation. This book provides innovative tools to help you understand and address many of these non-caloric considerations in order to transcend calorie math and enjoy practical and permanent weight loss."

—Jonathan Bailor, CEO, SANESolution.com, *New York Times* best-selling author of *The Calorie Myth*

"I love Jon Gabriel's visualizations. They've become an integral part of my morning routine. I now start my day with the framework only he can provide that includes gratitude, focus, and clarifying my daily intentions—all guided by his loving voice."

—Khaliah Ali, daughter of boxing legend Muhammad Ali, best-selling author, designer, and spokesperson

"Jon Gabriel is one of the most important voices in the nutrition and weight-loss universe. Get ready for a diet book that's unlike any other. He's written a unique, informative, and easy-to-read guide for working with weight. You're going to come away with a ton of great strategies and insights, all wrapped in a truly holistic approach. Highly recommended."

—Marc David, best-selling author and founder of the Institute for the Psychology of Eating

"In my functional medicine and anti-aging medical practice, weight loss is one of the most challenging issues I address with my patients. In 30 years I had never met anyone who has successfully lost over 200 pounds and kept it off permanently until I met Jon Gabriel. When Jon talks about weight loss, I wholeheartedly believe him. He is living, breathing proof of what works."

—Howard Liebowitz, M.D., FACEP, director of Liebowitz Longevity Medicine

"This book is created out of Jon's relentless search for remarkable transformation. You will feel he is talking directly to you with the insight and compassion that can only come when someone has walked the path. This is the go-to book for understanding how to harness your personal power to find your perfect natural weight without harsh dieting."

—Julie Daniluk, R.H.N., TV host, nutritionist, and best-selling author of *Slimming Meals That Heal*

"The most powerful healers are those who have healed themselves. Jon Gabriel has written the best book on weight loss, period. His work deals with the problem rather than the symptom and invites you to resolve the causes and conditions that contribute to obesity. He's not selling magic potions, quick fixes, or questionable promises. He offers an opportunity to find the wellspring of power in yourself."

—Frank Ferrante, star of the documentary *May I Be Frank*, featured in *Hungry For Change*, international speaker, and author of *May I Be Frank*

"With *Visualization for Weight Loss* Jon taps into a secret weapon that we all have: the power of the mind. We have personally experienced the amazing power of visualization and highly recommend this book to everyone."

—Jayson and Mira Calton, authors of *Rich Food, Poor Food* and *Naked Calories,* and creators of Nutreince: The Multivitamin Reinvented

"Jon's ability to connect the visible and invisible through the process of visualization is profound. His approach to body transformation and optimal health is truly unique and acknowledges one of the most powerful connections known to man, that of the mind and the body. This book is your ultimate guide to visualizing and creating the body and health of your dreams!"

—James Colquhoun, filmmaker of *Food Matters* and *Hungry for Change,* best-selling author of *Hungry for Change,* and founder of FMTV

"Jon Gabriel is one of the most conscious, authentic leaders of our time. His visualizations heal the root cause of weight gain. If you've tried everything else and nothing's worked, I highly suggest you read this book."

—Brittany Watkins, founder of The Watkins Method of Tapping for Weight Loss

"In a world where counting calories and strict diets have a huge failure rate, we need a new shift in our thinking, and Jon has written a much-needed book. This fantastic book is a paradigm shift in weight loss and body health."

—Donna Schwenk, author and founder of Cultured Food Life

"Beyond making conscious choices, losing weight permanently requires change on deeper levels that can be accomplished through the power of visualization. In this book you'll learn how to feel profoundly safe and relaxed so that extra weight can easily melt away. Jon shows you how to awaken your intuition so that making healthy choices becomes second nature, and slimming down becomes a piece of cake."

—Jena la Flamme, author of *Pleasurable Weight Loss*

"Jon communicates high-level spiritual and scientific information in a way that is not only accessible but enjoyable to read. This book gives you solid tools to turn on the mission control center in your mind so you can create a body and a life you adore."

—Emily Fletcher, founder of Ziva Meditation

ALSO BY JON GABRIEL

Books

The Gabriel Method: The Revolutionary Diet-Free Way to Totally Transform Your Body

Fit Kids Revolution: The Parent's Diet-Free Guide to Raising Healthy & Fit Children, with Patricia A. Ronald Riba, M.D.

The Gabriel Method Recipe Book: Lose Weight Without Dieting, with Oona Mansour

CDs & DVDs

Cellular Wisdom

Gabriel Method Fitness

Heal Your Digestion

Living Goddess

Living Warrior

Mental Secrets (Morning & Evening Visualizations)

Mind-Body Weight Loss Summit

Start Your Transformation

Weight Loss for Kids

FREE VISUALIZATION MP3 AUDIOS

To complement this book, get three free visualizations for weight loss led by Jon Gabriel. Access your MP3 bonus audio files here:

www.TheGabrielMethod.com/visualization-bonus

VISUALIZATION
FOR WEIGHT LOSS

The Gabriel Method Guide to Using
Your Mind to Transform Your Body

Jon Gabriel

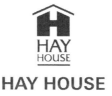

HAY HOUSE

Carlsbad, California • New York City • London • Sydney
Johannesburg • Vancouver • Hong Kong • New Delhi

First published and distributed in the United Kingdom by:
Hay House UK Ltd, Astley House, 33 Notting Hill Gate, London W11 3JQ
Tel: +44 (0)20 3675 2450; Fax: +44 (0)20 3675 2451
www.hayhouse.co.uk

Published and distributed in the United States of America by:
Hay House Inc., PO Box 5100, Carlsbad, CA 92018-5100
Tel: (1) 760 431 7695 or (800) 654 5126
Fax: (1) 760 431 6948 or (800) 650 5115
www.hayhouse.com

Published and distributed in Australia by:
Hay House Australia Ltd, 18/36 Ralph St, Alexandria NSW 2015
Tel: (61) 2 9669 4299; Fax: (61) 2 9669 4144
www.hayhouse.com.au

Published and distributed in the Republic of South Africa by:
Hay House SA (Pty) Ltd, PO Box 990, Witkoppen 2068
Tel/Fax: (27) 11 467 8904
www.hayhouse.co.za

Published and distributed in India by:
Hay House Publishers India, Muskaan Complex, Plot No.3, B-2,
Vasant Kunj, New Delhi 110 070
Tel: (91) 11 4176 1620; Fax: (91) 11 4176 1630
www.hayhouse.co.in

Distributed in Canada by:
Raincoast Books, 2440 Viking Way, Richmond, B.C. V6V 1N2
Tel: (1) 604 448 7100; Fax: (1) 604 270 7161; www.raincoast.com

Copyright © 2015 by Jon Gabriel

The moral rights of the author have been asserted.

All rights reserved. No part of this book may be reproduced by any mechanical, photographic or electronic process, or in the form of a phonographic recording; nor may it be stored in a retrieval system, transmitted or otherwise be copied for public or private use, other than for 'fair use' as brief quotations embodied in articles and reviews, without prior written permission of the publisher.

The information given in this book should not be treated as a substitute for professional medical advice; always consult a medical practitioner. Any use of information in this book is at the reader's discretion and risk. Neither the author nor the publisher can be held responsible for any loss, claim or damage arising out of the use, or misuse, of the suggestions made, the failure to take medical advice or for any material on third party websites.

A catalogue record for this book is available from the British Library.

ISBN: 978-1-78180-380-6

*To my father, the late Dr. Leonard Abrams,
who taught me visualization at the tender age
of ten years old. When I see the influence that you
continue to have on my life and on the hundreds of
friends, family members, and co-workers who love
and adore you, I understand fully the meaning
of the words "time loves a hero."*

FREE VISUALIZATION MP3 AUDIOS

Get Access to Three Free Visualizations
for Weight Loss MP3s with Jon Gabriel.

Get Instant Access Online at:
www.TheGabrielMethod.com/visualization-bonus

Jon Gabriel's guided visualization practices are used daily by more than 250,000 people from all walks of life, including celebrities, doctors, political leaders, athletes, and busy mothers. Guided visualization makes it so easy to commit to your daily practice. All you do is press Play, sit down, and listen. Jon will lead you step-by-step through these mind-body balancing practices.

Visit us online to access your three free
practices to complement this book.
www.TheGabrielMethod.com/visualization-bonus

CONTENTS

INTRODUCTION

How Visualization Helped Me Lose 220 Pounds

You've picked up this book for one reason: you've tried to lose weight and it didn't work. You probably think you've failed at dieting. You might think you failed the fitness trainers and doctors who have given you so much advice over the years. At this point, you almost certainly feel disappointed in yourself. Before we go any further, let me set the record straight. You didn't fail on those diets; those diets *failed you.*

The statistical reality is that restrictive dieting never works in the long term. If it did, we'd all look fabulous and no one would ever have to write another book on weight loss. Instead, month after month, some new diet appears, promising to unlock the secrets to shedding "10 Pounds in 10 Days" or "Burning Fat Like Magic!" No doubt, the authors and experts behind these programs have the best of intentions, but all diets are created around the same flawed premise that the only way to lose weight is through force, willpower, and restriction. Basically, you end up going to war with your body, fighting cravings night and day, and hoping against hope that you can somehow keep the struggle up for the rest of your life. The sad reality is that all diets have failure built into their very design.

Simply put, restrictive dieting doesn't address the real issues of why we gain weight in the first place, so it doesn't cure the problem. Sure, you can force yourself to lose weight in the short term by cutting calories or avoiding problematic foods. But if your body is forcing you to eat more or craving all the wrong foods, you end up fighting your body. Sooner or later, your body will win. You can control what you eat for a while, but you can't control how hungry you are or what types of foods you're craving. If you don't get to the heart of the problem, your body will undermine your efforts by making you insatiably hungry for all the wrong foods.

Rather than working against your body, there's another solution that is extremely effective: you can use visualization to get your mind and body to work together. It's an approach that's accessible to anyone with an open mind. The method presented in this book is a complete paradigm shift that delivers phenomenal results, and you won't have to struggle or deprive your body in any way. You're about to learn a holistic, mind-body approach that makes weight loss not only possible but actually easy and sustainable. Step-by-step, I'm going to teach you how to work *with* your body, rather than against it, to totally transform yourself from the inside out.

Why should you listen to me? I used to weigh 409 pounds. I was morbidly obese, my health and life were at risk, and the only thing I knew for sure was that I needed to find a solution. With my background in biology and extreme personal motivation, I became a fanatical biomedical researcher. During an 11-year period, I tried every diet—from low fat to no fat, from high protein to low carb, and everything in between—I tried them all.

I worked face-to-face with the late Dr. Robert Atkins (of Atkins Diet fame), who had me eating bacon and eggs for breakfast, steak and sour cream for dinner; in the end, when I failed to lose weight on his program, the best he could do was yell at me for being so fat. I went on to try the low-fat, high-carb approach under the supervision of the highly acclaimed medical team at the Pritikin Institute in California. When their whole-grain approach also failed to fix my problem, instead of throwing in the towel, I became even more fixated on finding the solution. I became a serial diet junkie.

I met with doctors, naturopaths, homeopaths, personal trainers, and nutritionists—and still no one seemed to understand that I was struggling with something much more complex than simply restricting portions or committing to an exhausting gym routine. No one seemed to understand that my body was fighting me tooth and nail, and the only tools available were no match for my cravings.

Every diet or approach I tried followed the same pattern. There was a list of "bad foods," things I couldn't eat, and I'd avoid them like poison. Then there were "good foods," the stuff I was allowed to eat freely, so I'd fill my fridge and my stomach with those approved items, trusting that as long as I did my part and followed the program, it would work. But it didn't. It never works.

The pattern was the same every time. I'd lose some weight initially, but after a few weeks (or a few months) on the program, my intense food cravings would completely take control, and I'd have a huge binge. Within days, I'd gain back all the lost weight; worse still, I would invariably gain a few extra pounds, adding insult to injury. This binge-purge, yo-yo cycle went on for more than a decade. It was one of the most difficult times of my life. When I hit my heaviest, my weight had become a debilitating problem in every area of my life.

Intuitively, I knew I had to address the real reasons my body was forcing me to gain weight. I just didn't understand why I constantly wanted more food than I needed or why I was so exhausted all the time and why I craved junk food night and day. So out of sheer desperation, I started using the mind-body practice of guided-imagery visualization. As a kid I'd experienced great results using visualization to resolve other challenges in my life, so I figured, why not? I had nothing to lose. Who would have guessed that the solution to my struggle with weight would come from something I learned as a ten-year-old boy—but that's exactly what happened.

As a child, I had terrible migraines. I would sit in a dark room for hours, trying to sleep while I waited for the pounding pain and nausea to subside. Painkillers wouldn't help at all and would only make me more nauseous. We were all at a loss over what to do. My father was a dentist and had developed a very powerful visualization practice he used with his patients for pain control during procedures. On a whim one day, as I felt a migraine coming on, he sat me down and took me on a mental journey to see if it would help. He started by walking me through a relaxation exercise.

He asked me to release the tension in my feet, my calves, and my thighs, until I had relaxed all the way up to my face and scalp. Then he said, "I want you to imagine that we're skiing at Waterville Valley," a ski area we used to visit every winter. "Picture yourself at the top of Valley Run," he said. "And now imagine there's a big bucket of black sand on your shoulder. As you're skiing down, imagine that black sand is tipping out behind you, sprinkling all over the white snow," he continued. "And now, imagine that the sand falling away behind you is your headache."

As my dad continued to guide me in this visualization and I had progressed to halfway down the ski run, the black bucket of sand had become half-empty. At that point he said, "Now your headache is halfway gone." And sure enough, my headache had faded. By the time we reached the bottom, the bucket was empty and my headache had disappeared altogether.

I was shocked that simply thinking certain thoughts and imagining certain events could have such a tangible effect on my physical well-being. I felt as if my father had just given me a tremendous gift and that I was introduced to something truly amazing, something that belonged to me that I didn't even know I had: the tremendous healing power of my own mind.

I soon learned to use that ski-run visualization to relieve migraines all on my own. Initially, it took me about 15 minutes to clear a headache with my dad's approach, but I later learned to banish the pain in just a few minutes. I then applied this healing technique to other areas of my life.

By the time I started my daily visualization for weight loss practice, I'd been unsuccessful at every other method of weight loss, and the situation was becoming dire. Part of the reason I was initially able to commit to a daily visualization practice was because it made me feel so good. But to my amazement, it did much more than just calm my mind. From the very first week I began visualizing, I felt an internal shift, and I knew I'd tapped into something truly life changing. Within a month, I could see some visible signs of weight loss. Then, like water falling off the edge of a cliff, the fat just started to fall off me, week after week, without struggle or force, without calorie counting or scales.

After getting into a deep state of relaxation, I would picture the body I wanted to have: a chiseled frame, defined stomach muscles, and tight skin. If anyone had seen the image I held in my mind back then, they would have thought I was absolutely crazy. I was 409 pounds, and there I was visualizing myself as a lean and fit 186-pound guy. As ridiculous as it may have seemed even to me, no one today can argue with the results.

Every night, I would visualize my goal, and then the next day things seemed to fall perfectly into place to help me achieve that goal, just like clockwork. My food choices started to change on their own. I wasn't craving junk food anymore; I started craving real foods, and I started having lots of energy. Suddenly physical activities like biking, walking, or hiking became fun again. I didn't need meal plans, diets, or exercise programs. My body knew what it needed to restore radiant health, and it all just happened organically.

Fast forward two and a half years. I'd reached my ideal weight and ideal body. When I say ideal, I really do mean it. I was 186 pounds, lean and fit. I was a living embodiment of the exact image I'd held in my mind during those transformative years. I had a chiseled frame and defined abs, and, to the amazement of my doctors, even my skin had tightened up to the point where you'd almost never guess I'd lost more than half my body weight. How was this possible?

Visualization is uniquely suited to retraining your body to be thin, much more so than dieting or exercise are, because it works from the inside out to change your biochemistry and neural pathways. I've learned that the biggest challenge in weight loss is not finding the perfect diet or the perfect exercise routine; the biggest challenge is convincing your brain that your body needs to be thin. From there, everything flows naturally.

I realize that the idea of using your mind in this way to solve your weight issues may sound highly unlikely—but I'd encourage you to keep an open mind. The mainstream medical community will likely take years to catch up to the latest research in mind-body healing, so the current diet myths will continue to linger. In order for you to break free from our broken diet paradigm, the most important thing to remember is that your body cannot and will not be reduced to a simple math equation. It is not simply about "calories in, calories out." I'm sure you know that some people can eat whatever they want and never gain a pound, while other people take just a few bites of ice cream and seem to gain weight immediately.

The types of foods you consume are certainly a contributing factor in weight gain, but what you feed your mind—your beliefs, thoughts, opinions, and emotions—all have a fundamental and overriding impact on your biology. It's your biology, or more specifically your hormones, that dictate how hungry you are, how much energy you burn each day, and how much fat you will store. Studies have shown that visualization works directly at the hormonal level to restore balance and encourage weight loss in natural and automatic ways.

We're now in a second wave of diet theory, one that emerged after the resounding failure of "calories in, calories out." There are new plans that talk about changing your body at the hormonal level. They recommend eating certain foods in defined patterns to reset your hormones. These are great programs, based on sound metabolic research. But unless you address the underlying stresses that are affecting your body's hormones, you'll get marginal results. It's a bit like driving with the emergency brake on: your body will resist you all the way. Dealing with the real issues—the stresses and inflammatory signals that increase levels of fat-making hormones—allows the weight to fall off much easier and faster, and *stay off!*

With regular practice, visualization will ease the stress in your body, and you'll build up the defenses to protect yourself from deadly diseases. You'll have more energy, and your body will once again regain the ability to lose weight easily and naturally.

In the coming pages, I'll explain exactly what's causing you to gain weight and give you simple, yet highly effective visualization techniques for addressing these issues. You'll learn visualizations that will help you:

- Reduce stress
- Create healthy habits
- Eliminate junk food addictions
- Resolve emotional traumas
- Develop stronger boundaries
- Sleep deeper
- Crave real, live healthy foods
- Regain the joy of movement
- Feel safer and more connected
- Increase your abundance
- Create more loving relationships

You'll even learn visualization techniques for activating the genetic expression of your "thin genes" and increasing the elasticity of your skin—all translating into easy, natural, and sustainable weight loss. Sustainable, because the real issues have been addressed and your body no longer wants excess weight.

Having lived through being in a body that once wanted to be more than 400 pounds—and that was fighting tooth and nail to gain weight—to now being in a body that is effortlessly fit since 2004, I can tell you that there's nothing easier and more natural than losing weight when your body wants to be thin. And these visualization practices work directly on the root causes of why we gain weight to get your body to actually *want* to be thin.

ıe only one who has experienced success with visual-
ireds of thousands of people around the world have
alization methods to achieve dramatic results—many
ıosıng - , 0, and even 200 pounds. These people, most of whom
have been on the dieting roller coaster for years, will tell you that
their success started when they began practicing visualization.
After suffering one diet failure after another, they are now fit and
healthy, without struggling and without being at war with their
bodies. Sure they eat healthier, don't have binges anymore, and are
more physically active, but it's all happening naturally. Their bodies simply *want* to be leaner. (Visit www.TheGabrielMethod.com/
success-videos to see amazing stories of people using visualization
to totally transform their bodies.)

The visualizations only take about seven to ten minutes
to practice, and you can do them yourself. You can also hear
recordings I've created of three of these visualizations at
www.TheGabrielMethod.com/visualization-bonus. Either way,
you'll be able to get tremendous benefits that increase on a daily
basis. Just like learning an instrument or practicing a sport, your
ability to visualize gets better over time. So if you're ready to tap
into a mind-body healing technique that's different from anything you've ever tried before, one that has the power to totally
transform your body from the inside out, let's get started . . .

CHAPTER 1

LOSE WEIGHT FROM THE INSIDE OUT

Here's a question for you: what do Albert Einstein, Oprah Winfrey, Michael Jordan, Thomas Edison, Martin Luther King, Jr., and Anthony Robbins all have in common? Besides being incredibly successful, they all credit a large part of their achievements to visualization. And it's not just these few super-stars. Tennis legend Billy Jean King was asked how she prepared mentally for a game. Her response—visualization. Nine-time gold-medal winner Carl Lewis would visualize himself winning before every race.

Visualization played a huge role in Jim Carrey's career, too, as he explained in an interview: "Back when I was broke and poor, I would go up to Mulholland Park, and I would visualize things coming to me that I wanted. I had nothing at that time, but it just made me feel better. I actually wrote myself a check for $10 million for 'acting services rendered.' I dated it three years later. Just before the three years were up, I signed up to do *Dumb and Dumber,* and I was paid $10 million to play that role."

Arnold Schwarzenegger also points to visualization as the reason for his achievements: "When I was very young I visual-ized myself being and having what it was I wanted. Mentally I never had any doubts about it. The mind is really so incredible. Before I won my first Mr. Universe title, I imagined myself walk-ing around the tournament like I owned it. The title was already mine. I had won it so many times in my mind that there was no doubt I would win it. Then when I moved on to the movies, the same thing. I visualized myself being a famous actor and earning big money. I could feel and taste success. I just knew it would all happen."

The list goes on and on. If you question the greatest in any field, from inventors to actors to athletes to politicians to businessmen, you'll find the vast majority have learned to tap into the power of their minds and use visualization to create amazing success.

In my experience, visualization is most powerful when it comes to weight loss. I can really identify with Arnold's words about how winning the Mr. Universe title in his mind meant he would actually win it for real. That's exactly how I approached my weight problem. As I was losing weight, I spent so much time visualizing myself in perfect shape that I had no doubt it would happen. It felt real, I saw it clearly, and then it happened. While most of my friends and family were shocked by my success, it didn't surprise me in the least.

The same is true for thousands of my clients all over the world. Sharon was completely bewildered by food choices. She'd tried a high-protein diet but got constipated and irritable. She tried going vegetarian but ended up eating too many grains and gaining even more weight.

"I had gotten to the point where it seemed like everything was bad for me except fruit and veggies," Sharon said. It's not uncommon for people to feel overwhelmed as they try to figure out what to eat and what to avoid. During our coaching sessions, Sharon wanted me to tell her exactly what to eat. She wanted a meal plan, but I encouraged her to take the focus off her eating and commit to a daily visualization practice. "Later, we'll talk more about food," I said. "Let's first start with the mind, and then the body will follow."

That's the inside-out approach to weight loss that we use at the Gabriel Method. It doesn't mean you're going to instantly, magically lose weight eating pizza and chips to your heart's content. But it does mean that by starting with the mind, certain subtle chemical changes will take place that will make you not *want* to gorge on junk food.

Reluctantly, Sharon agreed. She visualized herself being thin, picturing her ideal shape in a summer dress and sandals, walking along the beach. She imagined her hips and thighs thin and toned, the way they'd been in her early 20s, and she envisioned her chin and cheekbones sharp and pronounced as they'd been so many years ago.

Like I do with everyone, I asked Sharon to commit first to a daily evening visualization practice—nothing more. This evening visualization is one of the most popular visualizations we use at the Gabriel Method. You simply listen to it as you go to sleep at night. If you'd like to try it, you can download it for free at www.TheGabrielMethod.com/freecd.

The effects for Sharon were so immediate that she quickly started practicing in the morning, as well. "It's amazing," she told me on the phone after just eight days. "It's as if my cells are tingling in delight! And when I go out to eat, or go to the grocery store, I feel drawn to healthy, wholesome foods."

Sharon's experience is not unique. Many people experience similar changes. And while there's still a lot that science doesn't understand about visualization, the evidence is slowly mounting that harnessing the power of your mind will do wonders for your weight loss.

HOW VISUALIZATION ALTERS YOUR DIET

The weight-regulating hormone leptin plays a huge role in how much you weigh, yet we didn't even know leptin existed until 1994. It was discovered by Dr. Jeffrey M. Friedman at Rockefeller University.

As Friedman and others found out, leptin is produced by fat cells, and it helps the brain keep track of how much fat is on your body. Like most hormones, which are the chemical messengers of the body, leptin enables one part of your body to communicate with another. When a hormone is produced by one cell, it travels through your bloodstream until it connects with another cell somewhere else in your body, causing that cell to perform a specific action.

Hormones allow your pancreas to communicate with your heart, your brain to "talk" to your stomach, your stomach to convey messages to your liver, and so on. If you imagine that your circulatory system is the Internet, then hormones are the e-mails.

LEPTIN—THE MASTER HORMONE

Leptin is the master hormone in charge of body weight. The more fat cells you have—or the bigger your fat cells are—the more leptin you produce. When you have high levels of leptin traveling through your bloodstream, your brain gets the message that you have plenty of fat on your body, and then you stop being hungry. You get the opposite signal if you have very little leptin in your bloodstream: eat more.

Should leptin levels rise, a normally functioning body will realize there's too much fat on the body, and the brain will activate mechanisms that automatically trigger weight loss—and the operative word here is *automatically.* A healthy, functioning body that reacts to leptin as it should can lose weight effortlessly. Here's how it works.

When your body is sensitive to leptin, the way it is in thin people, your brain sends a message to your thyroid to produce more thyroid hormones, and that revs up your metabolism. Suddenly, you won't crave sweet foods as much and you'll have more energy and burn more calories. What's more, your brain starts tracking your food intake closely. Anytime you eat, your stomach produces hormones that indicate fullness; when your leptin levels are high, your brain becomes much more sensitive to these hormones, and you feel full much sooner.

Often, naturally thin people are active and seem to have lots of energy. You may notice sometimes they eat a lot and other times they may go all day without eating much. Or they may have all kinds of junk food on their plates and simply leave their plates half-full. That's the sort of thing that used to drive me nuts when I had a weight problem.

I had a business partner who used to order a burger, fries, and a chocolate milkshake for lunch. He'd take a couple of bites of the burger, eat a few fries, and leave half the milkshake sitting there on his desk all afternoon! I couldn't concentrate on my work. I kept thinking, *If I could get my hands on that milkshake, I'd suck the whole thing down in 30 seconds and get a big old brain freeze.* I was eating whatever low-fat, low-calorie, bland food I could find, based on whatever my diet du jour was. I'd eat everything on my plate as if it were my last meal, and he would be sitting there with a milkshake that was slowly, painfully melting all afternoon!

I'm sure you've been in a similar situation where maybe you're having lunch with a "naturally thin" friend and she'll leave half a piece of pizza on her plate. As she's talking, you can't concentrate on a word she's saying, because you know that if that food were on your side of the table, it would be gone in an instant.

The reason your thin friend isn't finishing her meal is because her chemistry is different. Her brain is more sensitive to the messages from her stomach. Leptin has changed the hormonal balance in her body so that she is full sooner, isn't as hungry in the first place, and burns more calories throughout the day thanks to her higher metabolism.

Hearing this, you might think a leptin pill or injection that would raise your leptin levels could be a magical fix for obesity. That's what many researchers speculated when Friedman first discovered how the hormone worked. To test leptin theory, mice were specially bred to be incapable of producing leptin; sure enough, these mice ate incessantly and grew to three times their normal size. Then the researchers gave the mice leptin injections. The results were just what the researchers had hoped: the more leptin they gave the mice, the more weight the mice lost.[1]

The next logical step was to give leptin to obese people. Sadly, the leptin had no effect. No matter how much of the hormone they gave overweight and obese people, they didn't achieve any lasting weight loss success. Even more puzzling for the researchers was the fact that their overweight and obese subjects already had incredibly *high* levels of leptin in their bloodstreams. That makes sense when you think about it, though, because the more fat you have on your body, the higher your leptin levels will be. Overweight people always have high leptin levels, but they're not losing weight. So what's going on?

As the researchers eventually discovered, obese and overweight people have something called leptin resistance.[2] This means that the brain is no longer listening to the hormone leptin. It's the same as having no leptin at all; you just get fatter and fatter. The cells fail to respond to leptin's message. To use the Internet analogy again, leptin is the e-mail, but the cells just are not reading them. The leptin e-mails are going into the spam folder.

With leptin resistance, even if you have 10, 50, 100, or 200 pounds of excess weight, your brain thinks you have zero fat on your body. And then what happens? Your brain forces you to eat large quantities of food—often high-fat, high-calorie food—so you can put more fat on your body. Then when you do eat these foods, your body makes sure that every extra ounce of food you ate, over and above what you actually needed to sustain yourself, gets stored as fat. Since everyone needs a certain amount of fat, your body is just working to get you to this healthy level—even though you're already above it. That's leptin resistance, and it's a living nightmare from a weight management perspective. I've lived through that nightmare, and unfortunately millions of people around the world are now going through this.

How can communication in the body break down like this? Why won't the brain respond to leptin and flip the fat-burning switch? You can blame it on evolution—and the wrong kind of stress.

FLIPPING THE LEPTIN SWITCH

In a research report on leptin from 2009, scientists at the Pennington Biomedical Research Center at Louisiana State University in Baton Rouge wrote that leptin plays a role in "powerful biological mechanisms that evolved to defend adequate nutrient supply and optimal levels of body weight/adiposity."[3] In other words, leptin resistance is something we evolved to help us gain weight for survival reasons.

Imagine living thousands of years ago during a long, hard, cold winter with barely anything to eat and no heating. That would be challenging, to say the least. It would be stressful. What would make that experience less stressful? More fat on your body. If you had more fat on your body, your organs would stay warmer and you could live off your fat stores until spring came. Fat is the body's natural defense against cold winters and famines.

Being in a famine or being out in the cold for days on end are particular types of stress that trigger specific chemical patterns in your body. These chemical changes are designed to make the brain resistant to leptin because being leptin resistant is the best way to force your body to gain weight.

That's all well and good when you're in a famine, but why do we get leptin resistance today when we live in a world of temperature-controlled environments and all-you-can-eat excess? The reason is because leptin resistance is triggered by a very particular type of stress: a chronic low-grade inflammatory type of stress.

We may not have to worry about famine and freezing anymore, but we still have stress. In fact, we have many more types of stress than we once did. We've got mental stress, emotionally traumatic experiences, toxins, processed foods, inflammatory medications, sleep disorders, digestion problems, nutritional starvation, sleep deprivation, and, last but not least, the stress of calorie-restrictive dieting. All of these can cause chemical changes in your body that are similar to the stress of a famine or a cold winter. Because these stresses produce hormonal signals that are so similar to that of a famine, our brains basically get tricked into activating the leptin-resistance survival program. So, in essence, the stresses in our lives are tricking our bodies into "wanting" to gain weight for survival reasons.

Your brain can't distinguish between the chronic stress of a long, cold winter and the day-in, day-out stress of trying to make ends meet, having an abusive boss, or dealing with other traumas in your life. You may not be facing a famine, but when you wake up every day dreading your job or dealing with a relationship gone sour, for example, the same stress channels are activated, and you develop leptin resistance.

WHY DIETS DON'T WORK

Once you understand leptin resistance, it becomes startlingly clear why diets don't work. Restrictive dieting mimics a famine. As you're starving yourself and fighting cravings left and right, you're creating the same chemistry in your body as if you were in an actual famine: your survival programs kick in and you become leptin resistant. The result is that you're hungry all the time, you're tired, and you probably dislike exercise. These survival programs are also why you might lose weight in the short term but eventually regain the weight plus more.

I call this survival mode the FAT—famine and temperature—program. The measures your body takes when faced with a shortage of food or with cold winters, such as leptin resistance, were originally designed to keep you alive. Now, they just make you fat.

Dieting is particularly harmful when your FAT programs are activated. Think of it this way: The part of your brain in charge of your FAT programs is called your hypothalamus, which is also known as your survival brain. Your survival brain is doing everything it can to conserve calories and build up fat stores. Some stress in your life is causing hormonal signals that activate your FAT programs. Then you decide to diet and start forcing yourself to eat less. Now you really are creating a famine. It's a self-induced dietary famine, but a famine nonetheless. This just reinforces your body's mistaken notion that you need to hold on to weight for survival reasons, and your FAT programs accelerate, making the body want to hold on to weight even more.

You hear it from dieters all the time: "Once I began dieting, I became *so* much hungrier. All I could think about was food." Well of course. Your survival brain is hell-bent on keeping you alive, and in its primal understanding, it thinks that eating as much high-calorie food as possible is the best way to keep you safe. The research report on leptin resistance from the Pennington Biomedical Research Center puts it this way: "Food restriction and fat depletion thus lead to a 'hungry' brain, preoccupied with food."[4] Essentially, successful dieting only makes you more likely to fail and gain weight. Faced with scarcity, your survival brain panics and takes more extreme measures to conserve fat. Remember, it thinks it's helping you survive.

Dieting isn't the only thing that can activate your FAT programs as we just mentioned: lots of chronic, modern-day stresses can flip the switch and cause leptin resistance, and we'll talk about all of them in the coming chapters. There are certainly things you can do with food to help address some of these issues. But those steps will be infinitely easier and yield far better results once you address some of the other stresses triggering your FAT programs. When you practice visualizations, your brain gets rewired for calmness instead of stress, and this reduces the inflammatory hormones that cause leptin resistance and activate the FAT programs.

We'll cover nutrition in depth in Chapter 14. For now, just a quick note; as a rule of thumb man-made foods usually cause leptin resistance and "real" foods usually help reverse leptin resistance and turn off the FAT programs. What do I mean by real foods? Imagine you were stranded on a tropical island—what would you eat? All the food naturally found on that island would be nourishing and would not cause excessive blood sugar spikes or inflammation. Real food includes organic, grass-fed, and free-range animal protein, raw nuts and seeds, leafy salad greens, veggies, fruits, and herbs. There are certainly exceptions to the "real food" rule, and we'll cover all that. In the meantime, try to add as much real food as possible to your meals right now.

Don't adopt a restrictive diet or count calories, but do try to eat as much of these types of food as you want. And if you're craving other foods, go ahead and indulge in them for now. You may not lose weight immediately, but as you listen to the visualizations and address some of the stresses that are setting off your FAT programs, your chemistry will change, and you'll find that you're drawn to healthier foods. You won't feel that overwhelming desire to stuff yourself with high-calorie junk. Instead, your balanced body chemistry will direct you to high-nutrient, high-quality foods, and you'll feel the desire to eat them in healthy amounts.

If you're currently on a restrictive diet, don't make too many changes initially, because you'll suffer a rebound once you stop restricting yourself. But over a few months, once you're no longer as hungry, you'll be able to transition off your diet and develop more natural eating habits. As I've said, once the body *wants* to be thin, weight loss happens more easily. But it can take some time to get to that place.

When you do get to the place where your body wants to let go of excess weight, losing it becomes virtually automatic. You simply crave less food, your metabolism speeds up, and you become more efficient at burning fat. Your body becomes more sensitive to leptin and other fat-regulating hormones. You become like those naturally thin people, have lots of energy, keep your blood sugar stable for hours at a time, go long periods of time without being hungry, and feel full much sooner.

This is the value of the inside-out approach to weight loss. By fixing the chemical imbalances within your body starting with the mental and emotional stresses, you'll naturally start to make better food choices.

Now that you understand why dieting *doesn't* work, and the importance of taking an inside-out approach to weight loss, let's look a bit more closely at why visualization *does* work.

CHAPTER 2

WHY VISUALIZATION WORKS

Picture a humble farmer. His name is Jeff, and he's just getting started with his farm. Jeff has only enough money to purchase a small field and build a 300-square-foot one-room shack with a bathroom. In his first year, his crops do well and he uses his money to buy more land and add a separate kitchen to the shack. The next year, the new land doubles his production, so he adds a bedroom to his shack.

A few years down the road, Jeff discovers a diamond mine on his property and becomes fabulously wealthy. Jeff now has the money to build an entire mansion from scratch. But rather than do so, he opts instead to continue to add to his humble one-bedroom shack. He tacks on a 13,000-square-foot lounge room, a fully equipped gourmet kitchen, and a 5,000-square-foot master bedroom with a sauna, Jacuzzi, and a heated lap pool. He builds a walk-in closet for his wife that is big enough to hold the clothes of two entire families.

All this he built around the original 300-square-foot room/kitchen/bathroom. It looks quite odd in fact: a sprawling estate built for the rich and famous all attached to a simple shack. Wouldn't it just make more sense, and be better integrated and more functional, if he simply started over and built the mansion from scratch?

Why am I telling you about Jeff's shack? Because the way Jeff constructed his house, tacking on a bedroom here, a living room there, is exactly how your brain is constructed.

THE BRAIN IS A REHAB JOB!

Jeff's original shack is a very simple structure—it's analogous to your survival brain. Your survival brain, also known as the hypothalamus, is a tiny part of your brain, about the size of a walnut at the base of the skull. It's virtually the same brain that a lizard has. There's no faculty for language or complex thoughts. It only responds to positive and negative stimuli—chemical signals that it monitors to determine basic physical survival needs, like how much to eat and sleep and how to manage threats.

The survival brain monitors how much oxygen you have in your blood and regulates your breathing, how fast your heart should beat, and how much sleep you need. It's in charge of most of your unconscious physical needs. It's in complete control of how hungry you are, the types of foods you're craving, how much energy you'll have, and how fat or thin you should be.

Eventually mammals further developed a structure known as the limbic brain—which was tacked onto the survival brain. This limbic brain's purpose is to process social cues and navigate social frameworks; it enables mammals to work together on a hunt or defend the pack from attack, and it helps members of a pack or tribe figure out whether they are leaders or followers. Dogs have a survival brain and a developed limbic brain. And just like Jeff's house, the limbic brain was built on top of the survival brain the same way that his first kitchen and bedroom were added to his one-room shack.

Primates, such as monkeys, apes, and humans, developed another area of the brain known as the cerebral cortex. This area of the brain helps accommodate more complex social interactions and allows us to ponder concepts like the past, future, and the meaning of life. The cerebral cortex is analogous to Jeff's mansion.

It is amazingly complex and intricate compared with the simple linear survival brain. And yet it's built right over the limbic brain and the survival brain.

Because of the haphazard way these brain structures were thrust together, the cerebral brain lacks direct lines of communication with the survival brain. You can look in the mirror and recognize that you want to lose weight, eat better, and exercise more, but your survival brain won't get that message. Just the opposite, actually. If seeing yourself overweight upsets you and creates stress and guilt about losing weight, the only message that reaches your survival brain—which is in charge of your body size and metabolism—is that you're under stress, you're threatened, and it's time to crank up the FAT programs.

Try this: imagine you want to stop eating chocolate cake and you say, "I hate chocolate cake." What happened? As soon as you formed a mental picture of chocolate cake, you then become hungry for chocolate cake and you start salivating. The salivation stimulates an insulin response in your body. And since insulin is the fat-making hormone, it puts your body into fat storage mode. All from simply saying the words, *I hate chocolate cake.* It's a serious communication breakdown that often triggers the opposite reaction to the one we actually want.

Basically, it's a problem we all face and we don't even realize it. *We don't know how to talk to our own survival brains.* Try talking to a lizard sometime and you'll get the picture. Our survival brain is in complete control of our weight. All it has to do is make some minor changes to the sensitivity of certain cells that monitor the fat-regulating hormones leptin and insulin, and the weight will literally fall off your body. And yet your survival brain doesn't understand a word you're saying. It doesn't speak English; it only responds to chemicals and chemical signals. In reality, just like Jeff's place, our brain would be infinitely more functional if it was designed from scratch. Or better yet, if we could figure out a way for our conscious brain to communicate with our survival brain . . .

How amazing would it be if you could have a conversation with your survival brain? What if you could say, "Listen, I know

I'm under stress and sometimes you get chemical signals that make you think I'm experiencing a famine or that I need extra weight on my body, but the reality is that I've got plenty to eat, I don't need any extra weight to be safe, and, in fact, it would be great if I had less fat on my body. Please turn the FAT programs off ASAP, please become more sensitive to leptin and insulin, and please lose weight immediately!" It would be wonderful, but unfortunately it doesn't work that way. Your survival brain doesn't speak English or any other verbal form of communication for that matter. However, it does have its own language that is relatively easy to learn: symbols.

SYMBOLS: A UNIVERSAL LANGUAGE

The power of symbols in invaluable. Let's say you've just gotten off a plane in some foreign country, and you need to use the restroom. You can immediately find a toilet because of the universal symbols of male and female that are on the front of the bathroom doors. Symbols are how we communicate with someone who doesn't speak our language.

The key to getting through to your survival brain is to use the language of symbols. You need to provide an alternative narrative to your survival brain, using symbols and images, that explains to your brain that you are safe, stress doesn't equal fat, and that your ideal body is one that is thin, fit, tight, and toned. When you use symbols, your brain understands and quickly makes the necessary chemical changes that allow you to lose weight. When you communicate with your survival brain using visualization, you're using the universal language of symbols.

When I finally began losing weight permanently, I started by creating the exact image of my ideal body in my mind. If anyone could have seen the image I had in my mind, they would have thought I was crazy. As silly as it might have seemed, I kept that image of me—at 186 pounds with defined stomach muscles—in my mind every night as I went to sleep. I felt a difference in my body from the first day I started practicing the visualization. It's as if my body just instantly knew what I was asking. I'm sure that from that day onward, my FAT programs got turned off. I had more energy, I wasn't craving lots of junk food anymore, and I was actually forgetting to eat and *even missing meals!* This was happening all on its own.

After I lost 50 and then 100 pounds, I was ecstatic, and I continued visualizing morning and evening with increased vigor and passion, until finally I became the exact image that I was visualizing.

If you listen to other people who have used visualization in similar ways, you start to realize this really can work. As I mentioned, Arnold Schwarzenegger has had tremendous success using visualization in bodybuilding and acting. Schwarzenegger also used visualization to *specifically* change the shape of his body. "I also used a lot of visualization in biceps training. In my mind I saw my biceps as mountains, enormously huge, and I pictured myself lifting tremendous amounts of weight with these superhuman masses of muscle."[1] If you've ever seen pictures of Schwarzenegger from this period of his life, you know exactly how effective his visualization was.

Gabriel Method students all over the world have experienced similar things; they know firsthand the enormous power of the mind to create specific transformations in the body. Rose began visualizing her ideal self when she was a size 22. "I had several chins, puffy cheeks, and flabby arms," she says. These were her targets when she created her ideal image: only one chin, smooth cheeks that highlighted her high cheekbones, and toned arms. Within four months she was down to a size 18. "My belt is now three notches farther in. I only have one chin, and my face is no longer round," she revealed to me one day. "I'm still losing and noticing big changes in my body shape—especially my arms, which have never before reduced in size with diet or exercise." For Rose, these successes are only part of her overall satisfaction with visualization. "I feel so good inside that I'm almost bursting out of my skin."

Cindy was battling weight and all the health issues that can accompany it: high blood pressure and kidney troubles that required dialysis treatment. She had taken her doctor's advice to restrict her eating and exercise more, but all that happened was that she got heavier and became more dependent on treatment for her health conditions. When she began visualizing, she didn't think about her blood pressure or kidneys, though: "Every night I would visualize my body exactly the way I wanted to look," she says. "It wasn't hard work; in fact, I was losing weight without much effort." Within a few weeks her blood pressure had dropped to a healthy range. In another month, her kidneys recovered, and she was able to stop dialysis. "Jon's method has helped keep me off dialysis for two years, and I've effortlessly lost 106 pounds."

Like so many people, Smita wrestled with low self-esteem. "I had struggled with my weight for years, and I had never been able to attain my ideal body," she says. "Until I tried visualizing, I had no idea of the impact a change in mental attitude could have." Smita began doing nightly visualizations, and after a few months she had lost 37 pounds. "I'm now slimmer than I was when I was a teenager, and I feel amazing."

One of the biggest concerns I faced when I was losing all that weight was my skin. Like so many people that are morbidly obese, my skin had been seriously stretched out. How would I get it to the taut, tight image I had in my mind? As I began to draw closer to my ideal, I developed a specific visualization for my skin that I used in addition to the one for my ideal body shape.

I imagined that my excess skin became a rose-colored glowing energy, and then I imagined a vortex in my navel and all the excess skin getting sucked into the vortex, never to be seen again. I felt my skin getting tighter and tighter. I don't know if this was the reason my skin retained so much elasticity or not, but the fact of the matter was my skin adapted so well that I had to get examined by a doctor just to prove to the publisher of my first book that I did not have any type of surgery. My skin was toned and tight just the way I had imagined it would be.

Is this really possible? Is it possible to use visualization to actually change the shape of your body or the tightness of your skin? I can't say for sure, and it's probably going to be years before we really understand the enormous power our minds have to affect the shape and fitness of our bodies, but if my results—or those of Arnold, countless athletes, CEOs, and all the Gabriel Method success stories—are any indication, it's clear we hold within ourselves a tool with uncharted healing capabilities.

When you unlock the secret of how to communicate with your survival brain, the sky is the limit as to what's possible from a health and fitness perspective.

SMART MODE IS THE KEY

To make your visualizations really successful, you must be in what I refer to as SMART Mode. SMART stands for Super Mental Alert Reeducation Training. It's an acronym for what brain researchers call the alpha and the theta states of consciousness. When you're in SMART Mode, your mind is powerful and relaxed. It is more open to making neural connections, and you can much more easily create healthy habits and implant your desired weight loss goals. In this state, you make a visual image of how you would like to look, and the consciousness of your survival brain can easily see the image and understand the message you are trying to convey.

So what is SMART Mode exactly?

There are four different wave patterns that your brain normally generates. When you're alert and working, your brain waves are in the *beta* state. The waves come in a frequency of about 15 to 40 cycles per second, and their amplitude is relatively shallow. This is the state your mind is in when you're dealing with the typical day—stressed out, frantic, juggling chores and work.

Next up are *alpha* waves, which are larger waves and range in frequency from 9 to 14 cycles per second. When you've just finished a task at work and you're resting, your brain slides into alpha state. Being consumed with a repetitive, enjoyable task such as painting or fishing, for example, can also put you in the alpha state, as can getting a great massage or watching a riveting performance. This is a reflective, calm place to be, and it's where your brain goes when you begin visualizing.

Theta waves are the slowest brain waves you achieve while still remaining awake. Theta waves have even greater amplitude, and they have a restful frequency of five to eight cycles per second. Daydreamers sometimes reach the theta state, as do long-distance runners. These waves are associated with the mind being calm, in deep concentration, and open to suggestion. Last is the *delta* state, which is typically associated with deep, dreamless sleep.

The key here is that the deeper states of consciousness, those associated with alpha, theta, and delta states, have higher amplitude, or larger brain waves. This is important because the larger the brain wave, the more powerful it is. The amplitude of an alpha or a theta brain wave can be 10 to 50 times greater than the amplitude of the brain waves we generate in our normal beta waking state.

Based on the calculation for the energy of waves, our brain waves are 100 to 2,500 times more powerful when we're in the SMART Mode alpha and theta states of consciousness. This means that any kind of visualizations you do in this state will be more likely to take. This is important when you're trying to break old habits or form new ones, which we'll discuss later. But it's important for all visualizations because you're tapping into the strongest tool you have for convincing your body that it's safe and ready to make a change. Brain researchers know that SMART Mode is where our brains are able to learn quickly, make faster neural connections, and create deep, lasting impressions. There are entire systems of accelerated learning techniques that are based on learning while in SMART Mode.

Also, your mind becomes much calmer in SMART Mode. Because there's less mental chatter, the images you create are clearer and more focused, so the consciousness of your survival brain is more able to receive the communication. It's a bit like looking at your reflection in a pool of water. If the pool is calm and clear, you can easily see your reflection. If there are ripples in the water, the image gets distorted. When you are practicing visualization in SMART Mode, you're creating an image in a calm pool of water, so to speak, so you are able to communicate your desired image more effectively.

When you combine the increased power of your brain waves in SMART Mode with increased calmness, you have the recipe for amazing change.

Deepak Chopra addresses the possibilities of visualization while in SMART Mode in his book *The Seven Spiritual Laws of Success*. In the book, he talks about two specific laws, the Law of Pure Potentiality and the Law of Intention and Desire. He explains that the Law of Pure Potentiality is a field of energy that you can enter that facilitates manifestation. If you enter that energy state, you are more likely to create or manifest your desires. That field of pure potentiality is the mental state you are in when you are in SMART Mode. Chopra explains that when you want to attain something in your life, like your ideal body, for example, you can accomplish this by bringing intention or desire into the field of pure potential. The vision that you create is the intention. So when you are visualizing your ideal body in SMART Mode, you are bringing intention and desire into the field of pure potentiality.

Again, we're years from knowing what's really possible when it comes to using visualization to lose weight and heal your body. But do we really want to wait the 50 or 100 years before mainstream medical science puts its stamp of approval on something as simple as our natural ability to communicate with our own brains? Already studies are coming out at an exponential rate that espouse the healing benefits of meditation and visualization, so I say why wait? The beauty of this practice is that if I'm right, and your mind really does have the ability to transform your body, then I've introduced you to a technique and an innate healing ability that you have that will change your life forever. But even if I'm wrong about everything I say, at the very least, simply by getting into the SMART Mode state and practicing visualization for a few minutes a day, you will be reducing stress and rewiring your brain to generate feelings of safety and connectedness, and just that little bit will make it infinitely easier for you to lose weight and heal your body. There's no downside, no side effects, and no risk. All scenarios are win-win. It's just a question of how much and how far you are willing to go with your mind-body connection.

In Chapter 12, I'll lead you through various ways to get into SMART Mode—plus how to create your own visualizations—but right now, I'm going to teach you one of my favorite ways to reach this powerful state—a simple way to place awareness into your body and use visual imagery to relax all the different parts of your body. It's called the "Ocean of Light" visualization, and it's one of the most effective techniques I've developed for quickly and easily getting into the alpha and theta brain states. Because all the visualizations in this book start with getting into SMART Mode, you can use this as you read the book. However, if this doesn't feel right to you, you can jump to Chapter 12 and explore other ways to access SMART Mode.

THE OCEAN OF LIGHT VISUALIZATION FOR GETTING INTO SMART MODE

(Note: This is taken from an actual guided, live visualization. The casual language and occasional redundant statements are intentional as they help create the ideal meditative state.)

> While sitting up straight, take a deep breath in; then let the breath out and relax. Imagine that there's a bright ball of bright white light circulating around your navel. Maybe it's the size of a large softball or a volleyball. And it's just circulating around your navel like a spiral or vortex of light. Just beautiful, bright, healing white light. And as it's circulating around your navel, it's getting brighter and brighter. And as this beautiful bright ball of white light is circulating around your navel, I'd like you to also imagine that you're in an infinite ocean of beautiful, bright, healing white light. It's an infinite ocean, as far as you can possibly see in all directions, of bright white healing light. And this light has the power to heal your body.

Imagine that, as you're sitting there in this ocean of bright white light, the pores of your skin open up and this bright white healing light comes rushing into your body from all directions. It's covering your body, energizing your body, and filling your body with bright white light. You can feel bright white light rushing into your torso, your chest, your neck, your head, and your arms and legs. You can feel this bright white healing light rushing into the bones of your body, filling your bones with bright white, vibrant life force energy. So the bones in your arms and in your legs and all over your body, all of your bones, are glowing with bright white light. And your muscles are glowing with bright white light, and your organs are being filled with bright, healing, energizing light. Imagine the ocean of energy filling your chest and your lungs with light; feel it going into your stomach and digestive tract. See the energy filling your liver, kidneys, spleen, pancreas, gall bladder, and entire torso with bright white healing light.

Now imagine the energy going into your heart and filling your heart with healing bright white light. And as your heart is filled with bright white light, it energizes the blood that passes through your heart. So supercharged, bright, glowing blood is circulating through your body now, from your left side to your right, filling every cell of your body with a luminous, glowing, healing energy. And you can now imagine every cell of your body glowing with beautiful bright white healing energy.

If you'd like, you can try recording this or any other visualization in the book so you can guide yourself through it. When recording, read the visualization slowly and calmly. The entire practice should take about three to five minutes. If you want to try it without audio guidance, don't worry about remembering it word for word; just get the basic concept of the light entering your body and spreading all over, healing and revitalizing, and spend three to five minutes practicing it.

Also, don't worry if it seems like too much to practice on your own. I've recorded three of the visualizations in this book, and you can listen to them at www.TheGabrielMethod .com/visualization-bonus. The visualizations we've created have soothing music in the background engineered specifically for enabling your brain to enter SMART Mode automatically. In fact, even if you didn't listen to any of the words of the visualization, you would still enter SMART Mode. So it can really be as simple as pressing Play and relaxing.

After you've reached SMART Mode, you should start to feel calmer and more relaxed and ready to imagine your ideal body or whatever your desired change may be. The more you practice getting into this state, the easier it will be.

Now, let's talk about how to specifically use visualization to address the real issues that can cause us to gain weight, starting with one of the most ignored yet influential things that packs on the pounds—stress!

CHAPTER 3

MELT STRESS, MELT FAT

Hannah was living in the U.K. and watching her weight climb. "My weight had been an issue for years. And stress was always behind it," she says. She tried a full life makeover by moving to New Zealand and taking up a new job. But within four years, the stress was back. "The work wasn't ideal, and I was living a life that wasn't suited to me."

As Hannah continued to gain weight, she began to develop other problems that go hand in hand with chronic stress. She contracted a lung infection, she couldn't sleep, and she began having symptoms of lupus and rheumatoid arthritis.

Understandably, Hannah succumbed to depression. Then, in 2009, she discovered visualization through the Gabriel Method. "I felt the stress easing almost immediately," she says. Even though she remained in the same job, Hannah began sleeping better. Eight months later, her lung problems cleared up, the autoimmune symptoms disappeared, and her stress levels were under control. Hannah also managed to shed 30 pounds. Now, four years later, Hannah has kept the weight off. Even better, she's managed to control her stress and prevent it from forcing her body to pile on pounds.

CAN STRESS REALLY MAKE YOU FAT?

Stress raises blood pressure, causes cold sweats, and keeps us up at night. But does it really pack on the pounds? Without question, according to nearly 80 years of research. As far back as 1936, in the science journal *Nature*, researchers reported that rats that were placed in stressful situations gained weight—especially fat—compared with rats who weren't exposed to any stress at all, even though both groups of rats consumed the same amount of calories.[1]

Much more recently, researchers at Wake Forest University in Winston-Salem, North Carolina, tried feeding monkeys a typical modern American diet. In groups, monkeys tend to have a well-defined social order, so the researchers watched how all the monkeys fared on the diet, with a special focus on those with lower social status. The idea being that the monkeys with lower social status experience more stress. While all the monkeys gained weight on the diet, the primates who were low in the pecking order put on many more pounds than those with the most social status. And the weight they gained tended to accumulate around the midsection.[2]

In 2009, a landmark study from Harvard Medical School clearly implicated chronic stress as a source of weight gain in humans. Stress researchers tracked 1,355 men and women for nine years, carefully recording their weight along with various types of pressure. They looked at finances, relationships, work—they recorded every potential stressor and compared them to the volunteers' weights. By the end of the study, the researchers had found that chronic stress could add 10 to 20 pounds on average. For men and women, the factors most strongly linked to weight gain included having little authority at work, little control over decision making, and a job that was too demanding. Difficulty paying bills was also linked to stress-related weight gain. In addition, women added pounds when their stress stemmed from feeling trapped in their lives or in strained marriages.[3]

STRESS ALTERS THE WAY YOU EAT

Battling constant stress spurs unhealthy eating, researchers have found. At the University of California in San Francisco, stress researcher Elissa Epel discovered that people have cravings for junk food when they're feeling pressure. Epel queried 59 women about stress levels in their lives and rated the quantity of daily stress they experienced. Women who were among the most stressed not only had more abdominal fat than women who were less stressed, but they were also far more likely to seek out foods that are high in fat and starch, such as donuts, french fries, and other types of junk food.[4]

So stress leads to hormonal changes that cause weight gain. And being overweight can cause stress, leading to even more weight gain. This is a vicious cycle that adds more and more pounds. Unfortunately, the next step most people take makes things even worse: they go on a diet. And as you already know, dieting just plunges your body into a state where it holds on to weight. Restricting calories just leads your body to produce more of the stress hormone cortisol, makes you hungrier, and eventually creates more weight gain when you succumb to your cravings. At the University of Pennsylvania, Tracy Bale, Ph.D., tracked eating behaviors, hormones, and genetic changes in mice on a restricted-calorie plan. After just three weeks, the mice not only had higher levels of cortisol, as Bale expected, but their basic DNA was altered in genes that regulate stress and eating. Next, Bale put the diet group in stressful situations. The mice preferentially went for higher-calorie chow compared with mice that ate regular meals. Bale concluded that dieting actually reprograms how the brain responds to stress, pushing the dieter to make high-calorie, unhealthy choices despite their best intentions.[5]

THE VICIOUS CYCLE

The research surrounding the impact of the daily grind on our bodies is clear: we're stuck in a vicious cycle of stress, weight gain, stress, dieting, more stress, and even more weight gain. Focusing too much on these study results could leave you feeling hopeless, as if you're in an uncontrollable downward spiral.

But there is hope. You hold the key to breaking that cycle. Before you can use that key, you'll need to understand a bit more about how your brain and body work.

By now, you know that stress raises levels of the hormone cortisol and other stress-related and inflammatory hormones. This triggers your FAT programs, those evolution-derived processes that your body developed to help keep you alive and safe but now seem to conspire to make you fat. The problem is that your survival brain can't accurately evaluate the type of threat you're facing. It doesn't know that your daily worries are about your boss or your spouse; it has no idea that a scarcity of food is a result of a diet plan, not a famine. Your survival brain reacts to cortisol and other stress hormones, and it responds in the only way it knows how.

When you're under chronic stress, pro-inflammatory cytokines—a group of hormones—begin to circulate, putting your immune system on high alert and raising your risk of autoimmune diseases such as diabetes and rheumatoid arthritis. Blood fats known as triglycerides rise, and they can increase the risk of heart disease. Levels of C-reactive protein, a marker for inflammation throughout the body, climb. The result of these changes is that your brain becomes much less sensitive to leptin (as we discussed in Chapter 1) and insulin, another hormone that helps regulate fat.

Insulin is the fat-making hormone, so, as you can imagine, this plays a big role in your FAT programs. As your resistance to insulin increases, your levels of the hormone rise. That equals trouble because insulin helps convert the food you digest into fat, which is then sent to long-term fat storage centers, such as your stomach, hips, and thighs. One of the factors in obesity that researchers are only just beginning to wrestle with is that not all overweight people eat more than normal weight people. One of the problems behind weight gain is that an overweight person's body is programmed to convert calories to fat and pack it away thanks to insulin resistance: you could be eating next to nothing yet still be adding pounds because your high levels of insulin are converting all available energy into fat.

When you look closely at the physiology behind weight gain, you begin to see that, ultimately, it's *not* a problem of overeating. Diet experts and nutritionists have been declaring that weight is all about "calories in versus calories out." They claim that if you eat more calories than you burn, you'll gain weight. But let's face it—if dieting worked, there'd be one diet, everyone would be on it, everyone would lose weight, and that would be the end of it. There wouldn't be hundreds of diets out there all offering different slants on the same flawed premise that you can somehow force yourself to lose weight against your body's will and keep it off.

No, weight isn't only an eating problem: it's also very much stress related.

THE STRESS SOLUTION

Finding peace in our hectic world might seem like a crazy dream, but it's possible. Whether you're looking to manage stress at home or at work, or to find relief from the daily pressures of paying bills and commuting, visualization can help.

Helene was struggling with an underactive thyroid brought on by constant stress. She had been working with her doctors to treat her thyroid and was having little success. Her weight had climbed during this time, as well. Then she discovered visualization through the Gabriel Method. "I finally stopped fighting my thyroid condition and realized that my real problem was stress," she says. Helene began doing the nightly visualizations, and the stress began melting away. "I had started a new job. And I had left my husband, who wasn't really the right life partner for me, but I felt a lot of guilt and stress about that decision." Although these stressful life changes had crippled Helene, through regular visualization she felt that she was able to find her own true self again.

"I surrendered to the complications in my life, and to my thyroid problems, and accepted them as part of me."

After visualization paved the way to this acceptance, Helene's thyroid problems cleared up. Then her weight began coming off. "I can't believe how simple it has been, and how peaceful I feel," she says.

Helene tapped into a tool for deep relaxation that's been well tested against stress. When you visualize with the Gabriel Method, you're doing a form of meditation. We use guided imagery to put you in a meditative state before we even start the visualization. So, in addition to the visualization, you also get all the generic stress-reduction benefits of meditation.

The research on mind-body techniques such as meditation and visualization has been so conclusive that most major health organizations now recommend using them to manage stress. In some of the most trying environments, these methods have helped people relax. In 2013, a Dutch study at Tilburg University tracked 88 highly stressed people as they took math and speech tests. The idea was to put these people in high-pressure situations and monitor their heart rates, blood pressure, and cortisol. Half of the volunteers then took classes in guided-imagery meditation; then the entire group took the tests again. The guided-imagery meditators managed to cut their stress response dramatically compared with the other group. The guided-imagery group's blood pressure remained steady during the exam, and they had lower levels of cortisol.[6]

Nursing is a profession that regularly turns up on lists of the most stressful jobs. Nurses are directly responsible for the lives of their patients, yet they don't have complete control over their patients' treatments. When you combine high risks and minimal decision-making power, you get the perfect recipe for creating intense internal pressure. Australian researchers at the University of Technology in Sydney decided to see what guided-imagery meditation could do for nurses and midwives at local hospitals. They asked 40 midwives and nurses to complete a one-day workshop on guided-imagery meditation, and then to practice daily sessions for eight weeks. By the end of the study, the nurses who were using guided-imagery meditation had cut their scores on stress tests by half or more.[7]

Visualization works its magic by addressing the very core of your stress, a structure in your brain called the amygdala. When you're under chronic stress, the brain produces chemical messengers called catecholamines that head straight for the amygdala; this structure plays a major role in generating emotions, according to neuroscientists. In a stressful situation, the catecholamines direct the amygdala to produce emotions of fear and worry. In 2013, German and U.S. brain researchers working together found that guided-imagery meditation could alter the amygdala's response to stress. The researchers asked 15 patients with anxiety disorders to commit to two months of daily guided-imagery sessions while another 11 patients received standard stress advice (go to bed early, try to exercise more, etc.). As a comparison, the researchers also tracked 26 volunteers with no stress disorders. Before, during, and after the study, the researchers used MRI scans to measure brain activity in the volunteers.

Initially, the researchers found that the people with anxiety disorders had much higher activity in the amygdala even in neutral, or nonstressful, situations when compared with the healthy participants. But after two months, the researchers discovered that in both stressful and nonstressful situations the guided-imagery group had much calmer amygdalae. In other words, faced with the same stress that activated strong fear at the beginning of the study, the guided-imagery group had gained control over their anxiety. The other groups saw no such benefit. The researchers marveled that the patients had "changed the [brain] areas crucial for the regulation of emotion."[8] They had essentially reprogrammed their amygdalae to react differently to stress.

When you calm down your response to stress, you also reduce the flow of stress hormones and pro-inflammatory cytokines, according to U.S. researchers at the University of Wisconsin-Madison. They analyzed the ebb and flow of cortisol and various cytokines before and after volunteers completed an eight-week course in guided-imagery meditation. Sure enough, the mind-body technique slowed the release of cortisol and pro-inflammatory cytokines compared with the group that didn't practice these techniques. What's more, the guided-imagery group reported feeling much less distress and fewer of the physical symptoms often associated with stress. The researchers concluded that guided-imagery meditation could "be of therapeutic benefit in chronic inflammatory conditions."[9] That includes the most troubling chronic inflammatory condition—your FAT programs.

REDUCE STRESS, REDUCE YOUR SIZE

Now, you're wondering, can alleviating the chronic stress of your daily grind really lead to weight loss? The answer is yes. Weight researchers at the University of California in San Francisco set up a study to directly address the question of whether mind-body practices alone could produce weight loss. They recruited 47 overweight and obese women to learn yoga, meditation, guided imagery, and visualization—specifically how to visualize love for themselves and forgiveness toward others. The researchers took note of the women's eating behaviors, weights, stress levels, and cortisol levels. The one thing the researchers did *not* ask the women to do was restrict their calories. After four months, the women were brought back in for more testing. Not surprisingly, the volunteers reported less stress and a greater sense of contentment. They also felt more in control of their eating; women who were obese had demonstrably lower levels of cortisol. But the biggest finding was that the researcher linked reduced stress, cortisol, and increased mindfulness to a significant loss in abdominal fat. The women lost weight—especially in the belly—without limiting their calories.[10]

The idea that taming stress can shed pounds isn't shocking to Veronica. "I went from 238 pounds to 130 just by doing the evening Gabriel Method visualization," she says. "I was in a constant swirl of stress and anxiety about my weight and my life. Now I

look better, I sleep better, and I trust myself." Veronica'ṣ
ing better food choices, just like the women in the stud

You can easily take advantage of what Veronica aṇᶦ ᵗᴴᵉ ᵛᵒᶫ-
unteers in the studies above have learned. When you practice
the visualization below—or any of the other visualizations in
this book—you will be rewiring your brain chemistry and your
thought patterns. You'll be moving away from fear, stress, and
weight gain, and toward feelings of calmness, connectedness, and
safety. You'll allow your brain and your biology to relax and let go
of stress-related weight.

SIMPLE VISUALIZATION FOR REDUCING STRESS

While in SMART Mode (see pages 20–21), imagine every cell
of your body saying at the same time the following words:

Calm, calm, calm, I am calm.
Safe, safe, safe, I am safe.
Peace, peace, peace, I am at peace.
Love, love, love, I am loved.
Supported, supported, supported, I am supported.

You have approximately 60 to 70 trillion cells in your body;
just imagine all of them saying these words in unison. Then
imagine the stress just melting off your body and falling into the
earth. Or envision a slight breeze that just blows off any residual
stress that's inside your body. Then picture a current of healing light entering your body and washing away any stress, cares,
or concerns. Imagine any excess weight you have on your body
melting away also, and you standing there in your most perfect,
ideal weight and body shape, feeling strong, confident, secure,
relaxed, healthy, vibrant, fit, and at peace with your world.

Any of the visualizations you practice in this book will help
you reduce stress. Simply practice them for a few minutes a day,
and you will quickly start to become aware of a calmness that

permeates your entire day, alleviating the stress response that was causing so many weight problems.

While it's important to understand that general stress can encourage weight gain, I've also found it extremely helpful to look at one particular form of stress that makes the body want to hold on to weight: fear. Sometimes fear can actually prevent weight loss because it makes the mind look at weight *as a form of protection*. That is, for some of us, fat can actually make us *feel* safer in an "unsafe" world.

OVERCOME TRAUMA AND FEAR

What I've found through my years of research and work with clients is that sometimes the body uses the extra weight as a form of protection. In fact, 65 to 70 percent of the people I work with can trace their weight gain back to an emotional trauma. We've had tremendous success in helping people lose weight by resolving those emotional issues.

When I first met Susan, she needed to lose more than 100 pounds. She loved chocolate and was convinced that her addiction was causing her to gain weight; she wanted help breaking her sugar habit. After speaking with her, I immediately sensed the issue was not chocolate (it rarely is). There was something else. "When did the weight problem begin?" I asked. Initially, Susan said she didn't remember. "Close your eyes, and think," I said. "When did your weight problem start?" Then she told me.

"It all started when I was ten years old," Susan said. "I had an abusive babysitter for three years, and I gained an enormous amount of weight during that time." Despite all the time that had passed since the tragedy, Susan was clearly still carrying the fear from those traumatic years. Already, she was on the verge of tears. We talked at length about the abuse and the pain that it caused her, and how she used weight as a form of protection from her abuser. She recalled that eventually she gained so much weight that the babysitter stopped abusing her. Her weight *actually did protect her.*

Once she recognized the source of her trauma, she was able to use visualization to deal with her fear, and soon she was able to shed the excess weight. This is an extreme example of someone gaining weight for protection from a past trauma, but it's much more common than you might imagine. I've worked with hundreds of people who have been either physically or emotionally abused in the past who started, subconsciously, to use fat to protect themselves from a future attack. I've seen men who were bullied and harassed as children subconsciously carry extra weight as adults to feel bigger and more powerful. Without even realizing it, millions of people use weight to shield themselves from a world that feels unsafe. This was actually one of the sources of my weight gain.

When I was working on Wall Street, I had a very aggressive business partner. He always had me on the defensive—he really pushed my buttons. Our relationship actually dredged up memories of being picked on as a kid by an older, bigger bully.

The whole time I was working with my partner, I just kept getting bigger and bigger. Eventually, I realized the extra weight was making me feel safer. By the time I was nearly twice his size, suddenly I wasn't afraid of him anymore. I think in my unconscious mind, I felt I could just sit on him if I wanted to. I could squash him like a pancake. My size was making me *feel* safe.

This is what I call "emotional obesity." People are unconsciously using weight to protect or insulate themselves from the world. The source of these beliefs can be a deep-seated memory like mine or Susan's or stem from more recent trauma. Sadly, cases of childhood abuse greatly increase the victim's risk of being obese.

Using your weight as a barrier is instinctive, but you can overcome this crutch. In reality, my business partner would never have touched me. He wasn't physically violent; he was just an angry person. I came to realize that my weight wasn't doing anything for me. But because of my deep-seated fears of being bullied, I felt unsafe, and the weight made me feel safer.

Through visualization, I was able to create a protective barrier between myself and this perceived threat in my life. Once I was able to convince myself that I was protected, the weight really started coming off.

EMOTIONAL TRAUMA AND YOUR WEIGHT

Whether you dealt with an intimidating parent or something much worse, childhood trauma can leave you at risk for gaining weight. Recent evidence of this comes from Julie Lumeng at the University of Michigan Medical School. Lumeng combed through surveys that mothers of 848 children had completed when the kids were 4, then again at 9, and once more when the children reached 11 years of age. The surveys queried moms about 71 different life events that ranged from performance in school to health problems to relationship troubles, and asked them to rate the events from extremely negative to extremely positive. Lumeng also measured the children's weights and heights.

After comparing the children's weights to the moms' answers on the survey, Lumeng discovered that children who experienced extremely negative life events were nearly 50 percent more likely to be overweight compared with children who had more serene, untroubled lives. The events most closely linked to obesity risk centered on the family's—or child's—mental or physical health. The risk held true for boys and girls, says Lumeng. The severity of negative life events predicted the likelihood that the child would be overweight as a teen, she explains. "If stress is related to children's risk of becoming overweight, this could be a new focus for interventions."[1]

One of the more dramatic illustrations of the way early childhood trauma can lead to weight gain comes from the Adverse Childhood Events (ACE) study overseen by the Centers for Disease Control and Prevention in the United States. Researchers collected health information and childhood histories from 13,177 people between the ages of 19 and 92. All the volunteers were members of the same health maintenance organization, so the researchers had access to their heights and weights along with blood pressure readings, cholesterol readings, and other measures of health. When the researchers looked for specific mentions of abuse from the volunteers' childhoods, they found that two-thirds of the respondents reported experiencing some form of abuse. After checking the weights in this group, they discovered a history of abuse dramatically increased the likelihood that this person would be overweight. For example, those who said they were "often hit or injured" or were "often verbally abused" as children were twice as likely to be overweight compared with people who reported no abuse.[2]

Abuse is an awful thing to experience, and a natural coping skill is to put it behind you and suppress memories of the incidents. But a study from the University of Illinois at Urbana-Champaign suggests that it is important to do just the opposite. Psychologists at the university asked nearly 600 female students to fill out a survey regarding abuse, eating disorders, and their emotions surrounding the events from childhood. The psychologists found that women with a history of sexual abuse who suppressed emotions regarding the event were much more likely to have weight problems.[3]

My client Sarah had struggled with her weight her entire life. After exploring her childhood, she realized that her overly strict and intimidating father had made her feel threatened, and she understood that she was gaining weight to help keep him at a distance and to lessen the disparity between their sizes.

When Sarah came to me, she had been wrestling with her emotions regarding her poor relationship with her father for years. "Once I realized my fears were still an issue, I began addressing them directly in my daily visualizations," she says. Sarah tried picturing a barrier between her and her father; soon, she began to drop weight rapidly. "The more secure I felt, the faster I lost weight. I managed to lose 147 pounds, and it wasn't a struggle at all. The pounds just fell away."

BATTLING ADULT EMOTIONAL TRAUMA

Childhood abuse isn't the only source of emotional trauma linked to weight. In my experience, an abusive business relationship stirred up memories of bullying as a child. However, studies suggest that traumatic events that occur in adulthood can also spur weight gain. Divorce, the death of a child or spouse, or even being the victim of a crime like a mugging or burglary can also trigger weight gain. Research from the Kaiser Permanente Health Group in San Diego, California, found that, along with childhood abuse, chronic depression and marital problems were also linked to obesity: they found people began gaining weight soon after going through a traumatic life event. (Depression treatment, by the way, carries its own weight risks. This is an established side effect of antidepressant drugs, and drugs such as Lexapro, Paxil, Prozac, and Zoloft can trigger gains of 10 pounds or more in 25 percent of users.[4])

Some of the San Diego volunteers were remarkably self-aware, stating that they felt their weight was a "protective device." I've found that many people don't realize the purpose their weight is serving. Making the connection between being fat and being safe isn't immediately apparent, especially when you're constantly bombarded by messages linking weight to calories and exercise.

THE PROTECTIVE BARRIER

Why would you gain weight when you feel threatened? As long as you feel insecure, as long as you feel threatened, your body will jealously guard your fat stores; this is a survival strategy.

Failing to lose weight when you're fighting emotional obesity *isn't* failure. People fighting emotional obesity like to talk about how they sabotage themselves. For example, you may go on a diet or start to exercise and lose 10 or 20 pounds. Then you suddenly break down and go on a binge. Maybe it happens as soon as someone notices and comments on how good you look; you might look in a mirror and realize you're slimmer, or you might be able to fit into clothes from a time when you were smaller. Whatever the trigger, alarms go off and you feel ravenously hungry. But the reality is, it's not self-sabotage, it's self-preservation. The body is simply fighting to keep you safe by using a strategy that's worked before. For Susan, her mind knew that bigger meant freedom from the torments of her babysitter.

Sometimes it takes a while to find the real source of emotional obesity. For me, realizing that my fears were driving my weight gain took far too long—though I had my suspicions. Have you ever looked for something you misplaced, like your car keys? You keep looking in the same places: on the table, the kitchen counter, the bench top, your bureau, all the convenient places. Deep down, you're pretty sure that they've fallen under the bed, but you don't want to bend down to look. You just keep going back to the same places over and over. Finally, you get down on your knees and look under the bed and, *voilà*, your keys.

When your weight troubles result from feeling threatened or insecure, attempts to lose weight can feel the same as looking for your keys does. You keep trying various forms of calorie counting, portion control, and exercise. You try every diet out there. But none of these plans will work until you feel *safe*. You have to identify the source of those fears—look under that bed—and then find a way to replace the protection your fat is providing. You have to convince your brain that you thin equals safe.

TWO WAYS TO VISUALIZE SAFETY

As we discussed in Chapter 2, the best way to communicate with your body is through imagery. And you can use visual imagery to help communicate to your brain two things: one, that you *are safe,* and, two, that even if you are going through emotional hardships or suffered from past trauma, the weight is not necessary.

Rewrite the Script

One way to resolve past trauma is to rewrite the story. By doing so, you're able to defuse the memory of the initial event, so that it's no longer motivating your body to store fat.

Just as your survival brain doesn't know the difference between a real and an imagined experience, it also doesn't know the difference between past or present events. So when you imagine a past traumatic experience with a more positive outcome, your survival brain thinks the scenario you're envisioning is what actually happened. The key is to first be in SMART Mode (see pages 20–21), because that's when you can access your subconscious memories.

Here's something you can try in your visualizations to help defuse a traumatic experience that may be influencing your body weight:

> When in SMART Mode, recall the traumatic event. Now imagine a totally different outcome. If you were abused by someone, imagine that person getting smaller and smaller, until they are the size of an ant. Then flick them away with your finger as you smile and feel calm, relaxed, and centered. Then feel the excess weight melting off your body. Alternatively, you could imagine a protective guardian or helper coming into the scene and defending you.
>
> If your trauma stems from an event like a car accident, imagine the cars missing each other. Or you could visualize a huge protective hand coming down from the sky and lifting your car out of harm's way. Then imagine every cell of your body saying at the same time the words, "Safe, safe, safe. I am safe, I am safe." Then picture all the excess weight melting off your body while you feel calm, centered, and relaxed.

A Surrogate for the Weight

Often, past traumas tend to get relived in present relationships and life situations. So if your threat is currently in your life the way mine was with the abusive business partner, you'll need a different approach. You can use visualization to create a power-ful protective barrier around you that acts as a surrogate for the weight. This way even if you're not yet fully able to resolve the issue, your body doesn't feel the need to hold on to excess weight, because it already feels protected.

While in SMART Mode, try imagining a column of light coming from the sky and wrapping around your body. This col-umn of light can protect you from anyone and anything—noth-ing can get through it.

To make the image even more powerful, you can picture this column of light from a distance—before you picture it sur-rounding you. You test its power by imagining it's on a train track. Now visualize a locomotive (with no passengers) hurtling toward the column. When the train hits the column of light, the column is unmoved, untouched, and unharmed, but the train smashes and stops instantly.

Once you've made that association, place yourself in the center of the column and feel all the safety and protection this column gives you. Then imagine being in the challenging situ-ations in your life that cause you to feel unsafe, but while you're imagining the scene, also imagine that this column of light is around you and you feel calm, safe, protected, and relaxed.

As you imagine you're in the center of this column of light, feeling totally safe and protected, visualize the weight melting off your body. Then imagine that you're in your perfect, ideal body, inside the center of the column of light, feeling calm, re-laxed, safe, confident, and protected.

Another great visual image is a guardian angel. Instead of a column of light, or in addition to the column of light, you can imagine a beautiful 12-foot-tall guardian angel wrapping his or her wings around you, while the weight is melting off your body and you're feeling safe and protected. Not everyone believes in angels, but if they are part of your belief system, this is a very ef-fective visual image. I've seen many clients have amazing results simply going through the day imagining their guardian angels were there wrapping their wings around them.

Once you've created the visual imagine of this protective barrier in your visualizations, you can use it during the day in real-life situations. For example, when you're at the office and someone is being abusive or threatening, you can imagine that column of light or the angel surrounding you, and you will instantly feel safer and more relaxed.

These imageries provide a great surrogate for your weight. Whereas your brain once thought that you needed the weight to protect you, you now have another form of protection.

It's almost miraculous how quickly many of my clients lose weight when they've made this association. People who have spent a lifetime yo-yo dieting and feeling like "dieting failures" are able to lose 50, 100, even 200 pounds or more simply by practicing these visualizations. This is inside-out weight loss at its best, because it really speaks to the heart of the matter for so many struggling dieters. We'll cover more visualizations for protection in Appendix B of this book, so you can find one that works best for you.

My greatest weight loss success stories have come from clients who have resolved emotional obesity issues. To see videos of Sarah and many others who have had amazing life transformations by practicing visualizations for feeling safe and protected, visit www.TheGabrielMethod.com/success-videos.

Once you resolve your emotional obesity issues, it will be so much easier to stick to a healthy lifestyle and develop healthy habits. Remember: you were never really sabotaging yourself; it was just that your body felt the need to keep the weight on for protection. With that out of the way, you'll be amazed at how easy it is to create positive thinking patterns that will propel you toward greater levels of health and fitness. To make it even easier, you can once again turn to visualization for support.

CHAPTER 5

TAP INTO THE BIOLOGY OF YOUR BELIEFS

The tendency to think the worst about yourself is common—dismayingly common. So much so that we tend to dismiss the power of these thoughts, and we're barely conscious of the negative paths the mind travels on a daily basis. "I'm not very smart, and I'm probably going to get fired from my job." "I look disgusting in this dress." "I really don't have any close friends because I have too many issues." "I'm fat because I deserve to be fat."

If this book is about the power of thought—the *transformational effect of visualizing* a better, thinner you—then it should be abundantly clear how damaging negative self-talk can be. But don't take my word for it. Researchers have observed how thoughts become reality in various cultures and in medical studies. Ever heard the term *nocebo?* The nocebo effect is when you believe something negative will happen, and it comes to pass. Anthropologists first observed this in cultures where shamans would place curses. Having resided in Australia for the last ten years, I know about research documenting aboriginal medicine men in Australia performing a curse called "pointing the bone." If they aimed a sharpened kangaroo bone at a tribe member, that member believed so strongly in the curse that they would soon sicken, stop eating and drinking, wither, and eventually die unless a healer intervened.[1]

If you think self-inflicted harm from dysfunctional beliefs could only occur in primitive cultures, consider this: in 2012, German researchers at the Technical University in Munich published an extensive review of nocebo research that revealed the nocebo effect is thriving in modern medicine. Doctors influence patients' health and healing all the time with the language they employ. For example, overuse of terms such as *burn, sting, pain,* and *hurt* when explaining procedures significantly raises patients' anxiety and sensations of pain.[2]

In another example about the power of negative beliefs, we turn again to Deepak Chopra, the renowned healer and international best-selling author on spirituality. Chopra often references the story of a friend who went in to see a doctor, and, as part of a general screening, the doctor ordered a lung X-ray. When the images came back, the doctor found a spot and brought the patient back in for a follow-up. "I have some bad news," the doctor told the patient. "You have lung cancer, and you have just a few months to live."

Within a few months, the man passed away as the doctor had predicted. When Chopra was going through his friend's belongings, he found a lung X-ray from 25 years earlier. When Chopra held it up to the light, he saw that the exact same spot was there. The patient had lived with this spot in his lung for 25 years; it wasn't until someone told him that it was cancer that it actually became deadly.[3]

You may have said at one time, "All I have to do is look at a chocolate cake and I gain weight." Or maybe you think you're genetically programmed to be fat. I know I used to believe things like this. If you look at pictures of me at my heaviest, you would have to say, "He has bad genes. He's fated to be fat." But people who know me now and watch my eating habits would say I am one of the lucky ones programmed to be genetically thin. It turns out that genes are not the most important consideration. Far more relevant are the beliefs and habits that activate our genes. Positive habits, thoughts, and beliefs can switch on our "get thin" genes, while negative thoughts and beliefs activate our "fat genes."

Visualization is an amazing tool for instantly changing negative self-talk and creating positive thoughts and beliefs about ourselves.

While mainstream medical science is only just beginning to actively study the power of beliefs, it's becoming glaringly obvious that beliefs are at the core of healing, health, and well-being. In fact, as long as modern-day medical research has been around, an inadvertent measure of belief has been built into every well-designed study. While you may not have heard of the nocebo effect, you most likely have heard of the placebo effect. And the evidence is mounting that the placebo effect is much greater than we previously imagined.

So much so that Herman Koning, M.D., founder of the Dutch Doctors' Association for Biophysical Medicine and medical director of Medipoint, says, "If you think you have an incurable disease, if you think it yourself, you are right. If you think your problem is curable, then you are also right. It all depends on your intention [belief]."[4]

Let's look at some of the amazing results from placebo studies that have come out recently that led Dr. Koning to make such a bold statement.

PLACEBO POWER

What is a placebo? A placebo is a medically inactive pill or treatment designed to trick a patient into thinking they are getting a genuine medical cure. For example, a doctor might tell you that you are taking a pill for arthritis when in fact all you are taking is a sugar pill. The original purpose of placebos was to use them as a baseline comparison—a null effect—against which researchers could test the viability of "legitimate" medicine. The way it's supposed to work is that test subjects will typically be divided into two groups: one taking the actual medication and one taking the fake pills. Ideally the medication should substantially outperform the placebos, thus indicating the level of effectiveness of the medicine. However, that's not usually the way it works.

The effects of placebos have long been an annoyance to researchers. They're the ghost in the machine that skews study results—at least, that's what the experts once thought. Scientists considered placebos bothersome because the inactive "inert" pills were supposed to be *ineffective,* offering a null response with which researchers could compare real treatment. Unfortunately for the researchers—but fortunately for everyone else—patients who believed they were receiving treatment tended to respond even when they were getting a placebo. That's why researchers are beginning to study the placebo effect itself. If a sugar pill can produce the same result as an expensive pharmaceutical pill—which often comes with troubling side effects—why not just give the sugar pill?

An area of medicine where placebos have proven to be particularly effective is in the treatment of depression. Researchers hoping to prove the worth of St. John's wort tested it against an antidepressant drug and a placebo. St. John's wort did okay, about as well as the drug. But it turned out that the placebo did just as well as the drug and St. John's wort.[5] For the participants, *simply believing* they were being healed turned out to be an effective treatment.

Scientists in the United Kingdom and the United States have analyzed nearly all the research done on antidepressants and have determined that placebos are as effective as antidepressants in treating all but the most severe cases of depression.[6] What is truly fascinating is that the belief that one is being treated leads to *actual neurochemical changes* in the brain.

Canadian researchers at the University of British Columbia tested whether dopamine—a neurotransmitter related to mood—would be released if a patient believed they had been given a "real" drug, when in fact they were actually given a placebo. In reality, all the patients were given placebos, but the researchers told some patients they had a 25 percent chance of getting the real drug. Others were told their likelihood was 50 percent. The rest were told their chances were 75 percent or higher. This last group experienced a medically significant jump in their dopamine levels, enough to have a healing impact on their condition.[7] So for these patients, their minds, through the power of belief, had the ability to change their brain chemistry.

This is particularly relevant for weight loss, because all that has to happen in order for us to turn our FAT programs off and lose weight easily is that our brain has to become more sensitive to the hormone leptin—a simple shift in sensitivity to a hormonal messenger. If our beliefs can change the level of mood-altering neurochemicals in our brain, they can certainly change the sensitivity in our brain to fat-regulating hormones.

You can look at the power of beliefs to affect your weight either from the perspective of the nocebo or the placebo side—negative thoughts create negative outcomes or positive thoughts create positive outcomes. If you have negative beliefs about weight loss, you're using your beliefs and the power of your mind against yourself.

Let's examine some of the typical dysfunctional beliefs that can interfere with our ability to lose weight.

It's My Genetics

When I was working on Wall Street and weighed more than 400 pounds, people would look at me and assume that I was genetically programmed to be fat. I was huge even though I didn't always eat that much. I also come from a family that struggles with weight, so genetics were an obvious guess.

If you've always harbored the assumption that you were born to be fat, you're using the power of your beliefs against yourself. Your parents might be overweight; maybe your siblings have their own struggles with eating. Whatever the source of your beliefs, if you assume you've been dealt a bad genetic hand, guess what? You'll be more likely to gain weight, and you will find it that much harder to lose it. When you consider that negative beliefs can cause pain, alter neurotransmitters, or even kill a person, then it's not too surprising that persistent negative assumptions could activate the genetic expression of your FAT programs and cause your body to gain weight.

What we're learning more and more is that your genetics represent a whole gamut of possible scenarios, but it's the expression of the genes that matters most.

The expression of your genes is triggered by environmental cues and signals, one of the biggest ones being your beliefs. We can see in placebo studies a wide range of physical and chemical changes in the brain and body based on beliefs. What's happening is those beliefs are stimulating the expression of different aspects of the patient's DNA that cause elevations in mood-altering chemicals and create physiological changes in the body. In short, your beliefs alter the expression of your DNA.

Dawson Church, Ph.D., the author of *The Genie in Your Genes* and founder of the National Institute for Integrative Healthcare, tells a story about a lady named Nancy who used visualization to help put her metastasized stage IV cancer in remission. She imagined little stars going through her body and puncturing the cancer cells and then water rushing through her body and flushing the cancer away. Church goes on to say that "filling our minds with positive images of well-being can produce an epigenetic environment that reinforces the healing process."[8]

Weight Loss Is Hard

Most people who have tried to lose weight by dieting and have failed time and again draw the inevitable conclusion that losing weight is hard or in some cases impossible. As I've explained, once you understand how your body's FAT programs operate, it's actually quite logical that diets shouldn't work. Every time you diet, you convince your body that you're in a famine, which causes your body to rebel and forces you to gain weight. I cannot stress this enough: dieting is a flawed concept that has failure built into its very design.

To me dieting is a bit like trying to walk through a sliding glass door. When you look at the door, you might not know the glass is there. It looks like an open door, but when you try to walk through it, you hit your head—*every time!* So naturally you might draw the conclusion that it's extremely hard or impossible to walk through that door. But once you slide open the door, you can walk through easily. It's the same with losing weight. Once you start addressing the real reasons your body is holding on to weight, you lose it quickly and easily. But if you are harboring the notions that it's hard for you or you're not meant to lose weight, those beliefs will get in the way.

My Metabolism Is Slow

I hear many people tell me that they have an underactive thyroid or their metabolism is slow or their hormones are out of whack. My response is always, "Your FAT programs are on, so of course your thyroid is underactive and your metabolism is slow." When you're leptin resistant and your FAT programs are on, your brain stops sending signals to your thyroid to produce thyroid hormones, so your thyroid and metabolism become sluggish. This is a natural part of the survival process when your body wants to store fat.

When you reverse leptin resistance, your brain sends signals to your thyroid to speed up and produce more thyroid hormones. Turn off your FAT programs, and the hormonal problems go away.

Even Hashimoto's disease—a disease in which your immune system starts attacking your thyroid—might be reversible. There are thyroid experts such as Magdalena Wszelaki and Andrea Beaman who claim to have had excellent success treating Hashimoto's disease by reducing stress, healing digestion, and eating anti-inflammatory foods. Together, these lifestyle changes strengthen the tired and overworked immune system, so it stops attacking the body's organs and glands. You need to develop a set of beliefs that support weight loss, and, just as important, you need a mechanism for instilling those beliefs so that they become *real* for you. This is where visualization comes in.

HARNESSING YOUR BELIEFS WITH VISUALIZATION

Marilyn Schlitz, Ph.D., president of the Institute for Noetic Sciences, was in a motorcycle accident when she was 16, as she reveals in *The Living Matrix,* a documentary on visualization and energy healing. At the hospital, doctors warned Schlitz that she might lose her leg. "I remember laying there with a cast from my hip down to my ankle and thinking about how to rally my immune system through my thoughts, such that I could promote healing in my leg." She tried visualizing her immune system targeting the damage in her leg in order to save it. "I could feel the tingling; I could feel the healing happening in my leg."

Schlitz's leg was saved, and, as she says, "I realized my mind was important to my body and that my body was important to my mind." She knew intuitively that her mind could help her heal. She used visualization and the power of her beliefs to save her leg.[9]

Webster's Dictionary defines *belief* as "a state or habit of mind in which trust or confidence is placed in some person or thing." These thoughts, habits, or patterns are stored deep in our subconscious. In order to change beliefs, we need to access the subconscious mind.

Hypnotherapists have been using guided-imagery visualization to relax patients, access their subconscious, and change their beliefs for decades. Hypnotherapists routinely use the process of guided imagery to change negative beliefs and instill positive ones. One popular procedure these days is gastric banding hypnotherapy: patients go through a guided visualization in which they're convinced that they've actually had gastric band surgery and that their stomachs are smaller and can't hold much food.

Stomach stapling isn't the answer to weight loss, and neither is "virtual banding," as this procedure is called, but it seems amazing that you can be convinced that you've had surgery by suggestion. Let's demystify this for a second: what is it that the hypnotherapist is really doing?

While hypnosis sounds complicated and mysterious, all a hypnotherapist is really doing is using guided imagery to relax patients and put them in the highly suggestible alpha and theta states of consciousness—SMART Mode. Once there, hypnotherapists can communicate more directly with the subconscious mind, where deep-seated beliefs are stored. They make the desired suggestions, and the patient's subconscious mind easily accepts them.

Making belief-altering statements in SMART Mode is an extremely effective way to change beliefs. And you don't need a hypnotherapist or anyone else to help you access this state. It really only takes a minute or two to change any belief you want. When you learn this technique, you become the master of your own destiny. You can easily create the optimal set of beliefs that best suit you, for health, weight loss, and life. People take beliefs incredibly seriously, but to me beliefs are tools. A functional belief can help me lose weight and be successful in business, relationships, health, and life, and a dysfunctional belief will only get in my way.

So I look at my beliefs in an impersonal way. If the beliefs are serving my life and helping me to reach my potential and live my purpose, I keep them; if they're not, they're out. It's just that simple.

CREATING NEW BELIEFS

When you start to realize how crucial beliefs are to your physical, mental, and emotional well-being, you can start to become a conscious creator in your belief system. Whatever the ideas are that you'd like to adopt, you can use visualization to program them into the very cells of your being. You can start to use *the power of beliefs* to your advantage. In a study conducted with hotel cleaning staff, the women were broken into two separate groups. The researchers told the first group that housekeeping was a great source of exercise and would lead to weight loss. The second heard no such announcement.

After 30 days, the first group had lost an average of two pounds, mostly in the waist and hips, simply because they believed their work resulted in greater physical fitness. Their belief led them to manifest it as a physical reality. As you might have guessed, the women in the second group had no change in weight.[10]

While a two-pound loss is not huge by anyone's standards, those two pounds were the result of a single 30-second announcement at a work meeting—nothing more. Their belief led them to manifest it as a physical reality.

Your unquestioned beliefs about weight loss are just as powerful, and they are getting in your way. So let's use visualization to help eliminate those dysfunctional beliefs and instill functional ones that we now know are true: losing weight can be easy, automatic, effortless, and sustainable.

Visualization gives you the handle and the key to open that sliding glass door we just talked about; once you slide the door open and step through it, the rest of your weight loss journey will be easy.

To help slide open that door, try one or all of the following three visualizations.

Weight Loss Is Easy

While in SMART Mode (see pages 20–21), picture every cell of your body saying at the same time the words:

Weight loss is easy, effortless, and automatic.
I easily, effortlessly, and automatically lose weight.
My body wants to be thin.

Repeat these sentences over and over. Imagine all 70 trillion cells in your body repeating these words in unison. Then imagine the weight melting off your body as all your cells continue to repeat, *My body wants to be thin.*

My Body Is Sensitive to Fat-Regulating Hormones

To improve your sensitivity to leptin, try this: While in SMART Mode (see pages 20–21), imagine the cells in your survival brain (the area at the base of your skull) have antennae or satellite dishes that receive hormonal messages. Picture more and more antennae or satellite dishes sprouting on those cells. As the number of receptors increases, imagine your body weight decreasing. See the fat melting off your body. Imagine your metabolism speeding up and having lots of energy and only craving real, live, vibrant foods. Imagine your hormones being regulated perfectly and the weight continuing to melt off your body.

I Am Genetically Thin

While in SMART Mode (see pages 20–21), picture your ideal body. If you already have that image, great. If not, simply look at a picture of your ideal body. It could be you at another time or a picture from a magazine. Just stare at it for about 30 seconds. Then close your eyes and imagine that image getting smaller and smaller inside your body. So small that it can actually fit inside one of the cells in your survival brain. Picture it going into the DNA of that cell. Imagine that once the image goes into the cell and touches the DNA, that the DNA strand vibrates as if to accept the new program for your ideal body. Then imagine that the message gets sent from that cell to every other cell in your body. Imagine that the DNA of your entire body starts expressing the genes that regulate your ideal body. Then imagine yourself becoming that image of your ideal body. See yourself going through your day, easily and effortlessly getting fitter and fitter. Then imagine the days, weeks, and months that follow and each day you're getting thinner and fitter.

Don't worry if you can't see these things happening; just imagine them or feel them as best you can, with the intention of communicating this message to your body. Your body will understand.

You can find more scripts for altering your weight loss beliefs in Appendix B. As always, if practicing the visualizations on your own is a bit confusing at first, you can always listen to the ones we've created.

CHAPTER 6

ONE BELIEF,
ONE CURE

In the last few chapters, we talked about changing our emotional states and beliefs to help us drop weight. And sometimes it's essential to address certain stresses, traumas, and other negative beliefs about weight loss—or yourself—to create the weight loss success you desire. But so many of us can't identify one particular stressor, one particular trauma or event, that has been shaping our lives. What I've found is that there is one underlying emotion behind all the things that activate your FAT programs: fear. And I'm not talking about any one particular fear, but rather a general belief that can make your weight loss efforts fruitless: the belief that you are not safe. Changing this one belief can entirely wipe out all the stress, fear, and negative emotions that we've been discussing up to this point. If you could program the belief that you are safe into your being, so that you never questioned it and it became an automatic part of your everyday life and your everyday thinking, the job of conquering stress would be done.

Our day-to-day lives are filled with challenges. Perhaps you have a difficult job or your spouse is distant and you're not sure where you stand with him. Your finances could be low, and making ends meet is overwhelming. Perhaps your children are struggling in school, and you can't see a way to help them catch up. With any and all of these situations, what you find is that you fear for the future.

Fixing each issue is one way to solve this problem. And certainly with visualization you can begin to become extremely effective at making the necessary changes to your habits and actions that will enable you to solve these issues. It's a worthwhile goal to tackle your problems, but it could take a long time to find a new job and a lot of counseling to fix a rocky marriage. By all means, look for solutions, but you need to manage these threats and find ways to feel safe right now—or you'll just keep gaining weight.

Consider this scenario: Two people who work at the same job and have the same position are waiting in a bank line to perform a transaction. Both are going to be ten minutes late for work. Both might get a little flak from their boss. One is able to put the situation in perspective and realize that sometimes it's unavoidable to be a little late and doesn't give the issue a second thought.

The other person can't gain perspective on being late. He can't stand the thought of facing his boss and the chance that he might get yelled at for being late. The stress escalates until he starts to panic.

Both employees are in the same situation, yet one is calm and relaxed and the other is feeling tremendously threatened. The stressed-out person is triggering hormonal alarms in his body; when he gets back to the office, he's going to need a cigarette or perhaps a donut and a bag of chips just to calm down. The only difference between these two people is that the one feels a little safer in life than the other, and the little threats and challenges he faces don't cause the same emotional trauma. It all comes down to safety.

So, what if you could instill the belief that you *are* safe? No rhyme or reason, no logic behind it, you just know and feel that you *are* safe. What if there was a way to change your perception of these problems so that they don't feel like threats?

CHANGE YOUR BELIEFS AND YOU *INSTANTLY* CHANGE YOUR EMOTIONAL EXPERIENCE

Imagine this scenario: You're sitting at a lovely outdoor café in a downtown plaza on a Sunday. You're waiting for your spouse to meet you for lunch. You've both been running errands and planned to meet up at one o'clock. She's running a few minutes late, but it's such a beautiful day that you don't mind.

However, 10 minutes turns into 20 and then into 30 minutes. Now you're beginning to get bothered. After all, your time is important and you have more errands to run; it's a little odd that she would keep you waiting. More than odd, it's a little rude.

Now she's 45 minutes late. The waiter comes by for the fifth time and asks again if you want to order. You say no and feel your face flush. You're growing furious. You think of all the times she's been late, all the times she's disregarded your feelings. This is so inconsiderate. *She must think she's more important than me,* you say to yourself. Your negative emotions churn, your stress climbs, your stress hormones surge, and your FAT programs are activated. You're not even eating anything, yet your stress hormones are causing you to gain weight.

Finally, finally, you catch sight of her across the street. She waves as she spots you, comes over, and plops down with a laugh. She talks about what she was able to get done, grabs the menu, and orders a drink when the waiter comes by. You're practically in shock, you're so angry. You're tight and short with her. *She can't even bother to apologize?* She looks up from the menu and sees your expression. "What's wrong, dear?" she asks.

"What's wrong?" you blurt. "I've been here for an hour! You think you can just show up without apologizing or giving me an explanation?"

She stops, looks at her watch, and replies, "I'm not late; I'm right on time. It's one o'clock right now. Daylight saving time ended last night, and we moved the clocks forward. Oh, my darling, did you forget to reset your watch?"

In a moment, your emotional world has flipped. You feel a wave of relief wash over you as all your negative beliefs do a 180-degree turn. Your entire emotional chemistry is altered in this moment, as well. Your negative thoughts are vaporized, and levels of stress hormones plummet as you realize, *She does care about my time. She is considerate of my feelings.*

What changed? Your underlying beliefs surrounding the situation. You were operating under the false notion that she was late, and that was causing a cascade of negative thoughts and opinions. The second that belief changed, all the negativity vanished because you realized that she was not at fault; *you* were at fault. Change your beliefs, and you *instantly* change the thoughts, emotions, and chemistry surrounding the issue.

Now imagine the same scenario, except there's no time change. Your spouse is really more than an hour late, and you're sitting at the table fuming. Your blood is boiling, your stress hormones are flowing, and you're inflamed emotionally and physically. She sits down, and you ask her in a voice that's quaking with anger, "How could you keep me waiting so long?"

She smiles and drops a brand-new set of car keys on the table. "Your birthday is tomorrow, and I just finished signing the papers on that BMW you wanted. It just took a little longer than I thought it would. Sorry about that . . . Happy birthday!"

How do you feel now?

The reality is that this time, instead of relief, you actually feel a wave of positive emotions wash over you. You feel your spouse's love and thoughtfulness. You feel warm—not inflamed—and you marvel at how lucky you are to be married to your spouse. You feel happy, secure, and content. This time, not only has all the negativity disappeared; it's been magically transformed to positive emotions of love, happiness, security, and joy.

Again, in an instant, you've dramatically altered the flow of chemicals in your body, and it's all based on your beliefs. Change your beliefs, and you instantly transform your emotional state. Take a look at the illustration on the next page—this is what happens when fear dominates in your life and you get trapped in a vicious downward spiral of negativity.

This is how a negative spiral can work in real life. You feel fear about something—your job or your finances, for example. Those thoughts trigger negative emotions (*I'm a failure, I might get fired,*

NEGATIVE SPIRAL

Fearful Thoughts
(I am not safe)

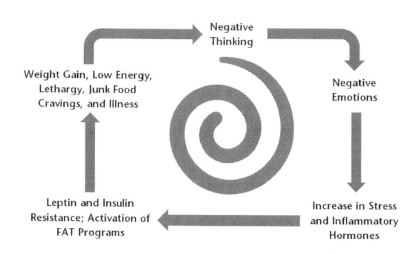

I won't be able to pay my bills, etc.). Those negative emotions communicate to your survival brain that you're in danger, spurring the release of stress and inflammatory substances throughout the body. Now your resistance to leptin and insulin increase and other aspects of your FAT programs kick into gear. You begin to gain weight, you feel lethargic, you crave quick energy in the form of junk food, and you make yourself vulnerable to illnesses like diabetes, heart disease, and cancer. Then you eat poorly, gain weight, and see your risk of disease rise, so more negative thoughts creep in (*I'm fat, I have no self-control, I'm going to die,* etc.), and the downward spiral continues into further negativity.

However, if you can change your beliefs—the basic premise in your life or in any challenging situation—to believe that you *are* safe, an equal and opposite *positive* spiral ensues.

POSITIVE SPIRAL

Positive Thoughts
(I am safe)

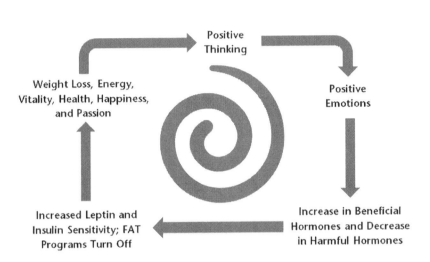

Positive
Thinking

Weight Loss, Energy,
Vitality, Health, Happiness,
and Passion

Positive
Emotions

Increased Leptin and
Insulin Sensitivity; FAT
Programs Turn Off

Increase in Beneficial
Hormones and Decrease
in Harmful Hormones

If you're able to feel safe, your train of thoughts will naturally be more positive. You'll experience emotions of contentment, happiness, and security; this will trigger the release of beneficial, healing hormones and suppress stress-related hormones. Your sensitivity to leptin and insulin will increase as your FAT programs will get turned off. This leads to weight loss, increased energy, vitality, health, happiness, and passion for life. As the weight comes off and your energy increases, you'll experience pride and more contentment, creating more positive emotions, and your upward positive spiral will continue.

The more you can create that automatic feeling of safety in your life, the more you can experience this positive cycle throughout the day. The ironic thing is that the more you feel safe, *the safer you are.* That's because you'll have fewer stress hormones cascading through your body, so you'll be healthier and less susceptible to stress-related illnesses, such as cancer, heart attack, diabetes, and chronic fatigue. And, of course, you'll be healthier because you'll lose weight. You'll have more energy for your job, which will translate into more income and greater job security, so you'll be safer in a financial sense.

You'll have more passion for your relationships and you'll be more conscientious, and this will help smooth out the rough spots in your marriage. People will be naturally attracted to your vitality and joy, so they'll be more likely to listen to you when you're presenting your ideas in a meeting or a sales presentation and they'll be more likely to buy your product or invest in your vision—all translating to more *real, tangible physical safety.* Simply by developing the feeling or belief that you are safe, you become healthier, happier, fitter, more successful, and more fulfilled.

So feeling safe will make you safer. You don't need a logical reason to feel safe; you just need to feel it. That's all that has to happen to reap the benefits. Sometimes this involves examining your core beliefs about how safe we are in the universe in general. This is tricky territory for many of us, because we're dealing with deep-seated beliefs. But I would encourage you to examine your beliefs about life to see if there's any way you can create a safer construct of the universe.

For me, I believe that the universe is safe and I am fully protected, both in this life and afterward. I don't care if my belief is true or not. If it is, great! If not, that's okay because simply by having that belief, I'll be healthier, happier, and more successful while I'm here. Either way, having the belief serves me.

Here are some key phrases you can say while in SMART Mode (see pages 20–21) that will help instill into your being the belief that you are safe. Use only the ones that you agree with and are comfortable saying, or you can make up ones that are more suitable to your ideals. Practice them in the middle or the end of your visualizations. Imagine every cell of your body saying the word, phrase, or affirmation simultaneously like a chorus of 70 trillion voices.

Use words here that you'd like to feel or believe are consistent with your desired belief system.

> *I am safe.*
> *Life is safe.*
> *I am on a journey.*
> *I am protected.*
> *I am supported.*
> *I am loved.*
> *I am taken care of.*
> *I have a place in this universe.*
> *I am learning about myself.*
> *This life is a beautiful adventure.*
> *I forgive.*
> *I let go.*
> *I appreciate this amazing life and the beautiful people in it.*
> *I accept all that I have experienced.*
> *I am always supported.*

Also appropriate here are religious affirmations, according to your beliefs, such as God protects me, God saves me, God is always with me, God radiates His/Her love through me. I am immortal, I am eternal, and so on.

Doing this visualization was tremendously healing for me. I practiced it for months. I can tell you that now, ten-plus years down the road, I just feel safer. I can't explain it, and I don't need to. It's just a feeling at the core of my being. As a result, I'm usually the guy in the bank line that's not too stressed about running late; I just have this feeling now that everything will be okay. You can very easily have that feeling, too, and when you do, you're nourishing your body with positive emotions all day, rather than creating a negative, vicious spiral, making it so much easier for the excess weight to fall off.

CHAPTER 7

PATHWAYS TO HEALTHY HABITS

When you adopt the habit of visualizing, you'll probably find that you automatically shed some other bad habits. Vinny experienced watershed changes when he started visualizing nightly. "I lost weight, sure, but every area of my life began improving." Along with making healthier food choices, Vinny also started drinking less. "I still enjoy a good wine now and then. I just don't drink as much because my body doesn't want it, and I don't feel the need for the stimulation."

Any bad habits in your life, like cravings or addictions, may start to fall away on their own once you start practicing visualization on a daily basis. That's because so many bad habits are coping mechanisms for an overly stressful life. When the stress goes away, so does the need for the coping mechanism. Nonetheless, you may want to develop more good habits to help speed up your progress. Whether it's getting regular exercise, improving your snacks by substituting fruits and vegetables for chips and candy, or watching less TV, good habits can make a big difference in how you feel and a big difference in your results.

I like to think of a good habit as an asset that pays dividends forever. The hard part is creating the habit, but once it's in place, it can yield positive results that affect every aspect of your life, automatically. You don't have to think about a habit—the behavior is automatic. Your morning routine is to wake up and brush your teeth, and this habit saves you countless thousands of dollars in dental bills and keeps your breath fresh and clean.

No one needs reminding how challenging it is sometimes to create healthy habits or eliminate negative ones. But visualization is uniquely suited to helping you add or delete any habit you want.

HOW HABITS FORM

What you may not realize is that your brain is specifically designed to form habits. They make your life easier. If you couldn't create habits, every day would be a horrific chore, according to Bruce Wexler, M.D., a neuroscientist and the author of *Brain and Culture*.[1] He has studied brain plasticity and how it plays a role in habits and changing them. One of the things he has learned is that we evolved to be creatures of habit. If we had to make decisions about our every behavior, we would quickly become overwhelmed. The brain's operating needs consume about 25 percent of the energy we take in, even though the brain represents only 2 percent of the body's overall weight. What's more, the brain expends 30 percent of its efforts in just keeping the body running—overseeing breathing, circulation, digestion, and other organ functions. If it couldn't form habits for which little brainpower is required, we wouldn't have lasted very long as a species.

To form habits, our brains rely on a neurotransmitter called dopamine. When you get pleasure from a behavior—whether it is something bad for you, such as eating french fries, or positive, such as performing well at your job—dopamine levels surge. This neurotransmitter then travels to two areas of the brain: one is responsible for memory, the other for desire, decision making, and motivation. The result is that the brain links a pleasurable memory to the behavior.

The next time you even think about that behavior, your body will release more dopamine in anticipation. Should you act on the memory and the impulse created by this anticipatory release of dopamine—you eat more fries, say, or stay late at work—the whole process repeats: even more dopamine is released, and this further reinforces your behavior. This is how we begin to form habits. The more you do something that your brain interprets as rewarding, the more you'll *want* to do it.

This dynamic is great for creating habits that have some immediate benefit because it's that in-the-moment reward that generates the dopamine response. However, it's often the bad habits that provide instant gratification, such as eating junk food, drinking, taking drugs, or watching TV.

How can you create good habits like exercising, drinking wheatgrass juice, doing homework, or cleaning your desk? These behaviors don't always offer immediate benefits and therefore rarely trigger that pleasurable chemical release that kick-starts the habit-forming dynamic.

The tried-and-true method for forming healthy habits is a little like drudgery: you force yourself to do these actions day in and day out until one day (hopefully!) they become a habit. Eventually, you create a neural network for the habit, which is like a well-worn path in the brain. These networks are long strings of brain cells connected to each other, like a winding path through a field. Picture a huge field of tall grass that comes up to your waist that you need to walk through. The first time you try to make a path, there are any number of directions you could choose. But the second time through, you're more likely to take the path you made the first time. Eventually, you'll have a trail of trampled grass that offers little resistance and requires little effort to follow.

Our brain works in the same way. The more times two brain cells, or neurons, communicate with one another, the more chemical receptors they develop at the interface between them. More receptors mean that it's much easier and requires much less energy and effort for the two cells to "talk" to each other. Doing or thinking the same thing over and over wears a path in your brain, and it gets more and more reinforced each time you repeat the action.

Traversing the well-worn paths of your mind—those established neural networks—can be fine if the habit happens to be a healthy one, but not if the path leads to a behavior you're trying to change. In that case, straying off the well-worn path and forging a new one will take a lot of focus, attention, and energy.

You may remember that when you were young, charging off in a new direction through a field of tall grass would have been easy and fun. You might have done it on purpose just for the thrill of breaking new ground. Not surprisingly, younger minds form new neural pathways much more easily. A youthful brain is more malleable or "plastic," a trait that fades with age. Once we're out of our teens, our brains lose some of their plasticity and ability to form new neural networks; altering the old ones can present a real challenge.

Don't lose hope. There is one practice that has been proven to restore plasticity and malleability to the brain: visualization.

CHANGING HABITS

First, you should know that going after bad habits can pay some big dividends. If this feels a bit daunting at first, remember Vinny's experience: simply by developing the habit of visualizing, he was able to suddenly form several new beneficial habits and shed some bad ones in the process. This snowball effect has been documented in research. In 2012, researchers at Northwestern University in Chicago designed a study on the beneficial effects of healthy change. They randomly assigned 204 people between the ages of 21 and 60 to try and increase their fruit and vegetable intake, increase exercise, decrease sedentary time in front of the computer or television, or reduce the amount of saturated fat in their diets. To get them started, the researchers promised to pay the volunteers $175 at the end of three weeks if the volunteers met their goals.

The cash incentive worked wonders, as nearly all the volunteers earned a payout. The researchers then continued to track the study subjects for the next six months, checking in periodically to see how their new habits were going. The volunteers were not only able to keep up their original goals; they began to add other healthy habits. Eating more fruits and vegetables led to a desire to reduce unhealthy foods. Cutting back on couch-potato time led to more exercise.[2]

The research indicates that tackling just one bad habit can have a domino effect on other undesirable behaviors. And since visualization is in itself a positive habit, you can count on several more coming with it. You'll also be able to use it to create even more positive habits—or paths through that field of grass—by increasing the plasticity of your brain.

Noted health and heart researcher Dean Ornish, M.D., at the University of California in San Francisco, recently completed an analysis of the brains of people who regularly meditate or do yoga. As I've pointed out before, the way the Gabriel Method uses visualization incorporates all the benefits of meditation. Ornish discovered that, compared with people who never practiced relaxation techniques, the meditators and yoga practitioners had much longer protective caps—called telomeres—on the ends of their chromosomes.[3] Telomeres shorten as we get older; when they get too short, cells die off. Over the past several years, researchers have linked shorter telomeres to a broad range of aging-related diseases, such as cancer, heart disease, and dementia.

In Ornish's study, the people who were performing visualization and meditation-related exercises not only had longer telomeres; they actually lengthened the protective caps by 43 percent over the five years of the study. They were essentially reversing aging in the brain, according to Ornish.

As we already know, a younger brain can more easily form new neural networks and new habits. When you use visualization to create positive behaviors, you'll be surprised at how quickly your intentions become reality. After sliding into a contemplative, relaxed mental state—SMART Mode—your brain waves become much more powerful, and your brain actually becomes "younger" in a sense.

Children spend most of their time in the meditative alpha and theta states, which is why they can learn things so much faster. These are the brain states you reach with visualization. You can regain the neuroplasticity of childhood and use those brain wave states to quickly create any habit you want.

Remember, when you're in SMART Mode you combine increased brainpower with increased focus and concentration. While in that state you have an extremely potent combination that can quickly forge new neural networks, allowing you to easily break bad habits and rapidly create new ones.

Employing visualization to create new habits is like using a bulldozer to make a path. Yes, walking through tall grass once a day will eventually create a path, but you can make a new path in minutes using a bulldozer. In the same way, you can create new habits and eliminate bad habits in minutes using visualization in SMART Mode.

You'll find this approach much more gratifying and rewarding than relying on the established methods of developing good habits through willpower and brute repetition, which can take months or years to really groove a new trail through your neural network. With visualization you can embed new paths and new patterns of behavior in a matter of days.

There's also another way visualization can help you maintain your new behaviors. In a study from Germany, researchers monitored the brains of 69 volunteers as they put them in stressful situations. The researchers found that under stress, goal-oriented parts of the brain shut down, while areas responsible for habitual behavior remain active.[4] What that means, as most people instinctively know, is that under stress we revert to old habits. The focus on the prize—your long-term goal of achieving the perfect image of yourself—falls to the wayside and you turn to the junk foods and destructive behaviors that give immediate relief.

Once again, stress can be poison when it comes to adopting new healthy behaviors and reaching your ideal self. Lucky for you, you're already practicing the antidote. Visualization will alleviate that stress and make you resistant to the lure of comfort food and negative behaviors.

Starting on page 70 you'll find a visualization that you can customize as you like. This visualization will help you instantly create new positive habits and eliminate negative ones.

But first, let's talk about the type of healthy habits you might want to adopt:

- Eating and loving healthy, live, vibrant foods

- Making a green juice or green smoothie, or taking a super-green supplement

- Loving your chosen physical activity and doing it automatically, without having to force yourself

- Taking probiotics and healthy supplements each day

- Practicing visualization or meditation first thing in the morning

- Being more productive at work

- Pursuing creative endeavors and being prolific in your creative expression

- Taking a warm bath and doing some light stretching or yoga at night instead of watching TV

- Always finishing your work before you leave the office

- Cleaning your desk before you leave the office

- Being more patient and present with your kids

- Drinking mineral water with lemon and stevia instead of soda or diet soda

- Doing healthy mind-body practices to de-stress and unwind instead of having a drink

- Taking a healthy afternoon snack to work instead of hitting the vending machines

- Spending more time reading and writing, rather than being on the Internet

- Going to a juice bar or raw food snack bar after work instead of a drive-through fast-food restaurant

- Playing in the park with your kids, rather than putting them in front of the TV

- Going for a family walk or swim before or after dinner

- Having dinners together as a family

- Learning new delicious, super-healthy ways to make breads, crackers, cakes, muffins, pastas, and desserts

- Serving healthy, delicious foods for your kid's lunch

- Learning to be more present, loving, accepting, forgiving, and appreciative of yourself and others

This list is just a starting place. You may have other habits that you want to focus on. For any habit you wish to create, simply visualize yourself doing the habit, while in SMART Mode, and then imagine yourself loving the new positive action and feeling tremendous benefits.

CREATING HEALTHY HABITS VISUALIZATION

If you'd like to create the habit of taking a family walk after dinner, try this visualization:

> While in SMART Mode (see pages 20–21), imagine coming home from work feeling calm, refreshed, energized, and present. See yourself preparing a healthy, delicious meal for your family. Feel the vegetables in your hand as you're cutting them, smell the herbs roasting in the stir-fry, and see how delicious and appetizing the food looks. Then imagine everyone coming home and sitting down together and having an amazing meal. See yourself feeling calm, relaxed, and present—giving your family all the love and attention they deserve. Imagine choosing healthy, live, vibrant foods at the dinner table, eating slowly, stopping frequently, feeling energized and satisfied, and having a marvelous time with your loved ones.
>
> Then see yourself walking outside with your family—walking slowly, calmly, relaxed, and smiling. Hear the sounds of the birds

chirping, the gentle breeze rustling through the trees, and feel the soft grass on your feet. Imagine that you're holding hands with members of your family. Feel your child's hand in yours. Imagine that you all are singing or laughing and joking and having a beautiful time just soaking up the moment. See yourself as you're walking, feeling happy, relaxed, calm, confident, centered, and totally focused on the moment.

You can practice a visualization like this for any positive habit you'd like to create. For example, if you want to wake up early and go to the gym, simply imagine yourself doing so as you are going to sleep. The mental rehearsal activates neural pathways as if you're actually doing the event you're imagining. Studies with athletes have shown that when they imagine their ideal sport, the same neurons get fired as if they are actually doing the sport. So when you imagine yourself doing something, you are actually activating the brain cells in charge of forming that habit.

I find I will be much more likely to do anything I'd like to do in a day if I first imagine myself doing the event the night before as I'm going to sleep. So as you're going to sleep at night or during your visualizations, imagine yourself doing the desired habit, loving it, and getting tremendous benefit. See yourself going to the gym, putting on your sneakers, tying your shoelaces, going on the court, and having an awesome game of basketball. See yourself scoring point after point, moving fast, feeling amazing, and loving every minute of it. Imagine waking up and making a delicious smoothie and loving the taste of it. Feel it nourishing your body and the weight melting off you. Again, these are just examples; the sky is the limit. By simply imagining the coming day as you are going to sleep at night, or during your visualizations—all the healthy, productive things you'd like to achieve—you'll have a powerful mechanism in place for creating those habits.

Now that we've looked at some of the bigger underlying issues that create problems for losing weight, let's dive a bit deeper into how we can use visualization and our newfound ability to create healthy habits to address some of the day-to-day issues we experience that can keep us stuck.

CHAPTER 8

REDISCOVER THE JOY OF MOVEMENT

Extreme exercise programs have reached a new level of ridiculousness. If you've ever watched late-night TV infomercials, you know exactly what I'm talking about. Gone are the days of "8 Minute Abs"; today's at-home fitness gurus now recommend one to two hours of grueling, military-style workouts that are painful just to watch. This "more is better" concept is meant to burn the maximum calories, but in reality it leaves most people intimidated, sore, exhausted, and hungry. Yes, that's right. Extreme exercise often leaves you hungrier than when you started, which defeats the whole purpose!

Let me be clear here—exercise is wonderful. I love to swim in the ocean, race around on my bike, and chase my daughter in the park. But when I weighed more than 400 pounds, I'd break a sweat just trying to tie my shoes. The days when I forced myself to go to the gym and pedal for an hour on a stationary bike were excruciating and miserable, and they did nothing to help me lose weight.

Thankfully, visualization is a great way to regain your love of movement. Forget about treadmills and stair climbing: start by remembering and visualizing the physical activities that you used to love—or anything that excites you now. I've always loved cycling. While it was impossible for me to ride my bike at my top weight, as I dropped some pounds I was able to ride more and more. Even now, cycling remains one of my favorite activities. Maybe you're excited by the idea of dancing, swimming, or hiking in the woods.

Whatever it is you love (or used to love), focus on that, visualize it, and you'll most likely find that you'll start being more active naturally.

Gabriel Method student Desiree had given up trying to lose weight. She had yo-yo dieted to the point of absolute despair, and, as she put it, "I was either going to lose the weight or lose my life." I knew exactly what she felt like, and I also knew that there was help.

Desiree was open-minded about my approach and right away committed to her nightly visualizations. Within weeks, she began making better food choices, like many people do, but more surprising to her was that exercise suddenly became fun and easy. After a month of visualization, Desiree started taking swimming lessons for the first time in her life—something she had always wanted to do but had never found the time or courage to pursue. To her own delight, she found she didn't have to force herself to go to the pool. She actually looked forward to it, and it became the highlight of her day.

To date, Desiree has shed 119 pounds, and exercise has become a regular part of her life by choice, and it never feels like a chore or a workout. Like many Gabriel Method students, Desiree discovered that visualization can lead to a spontaneous interest in physical activities, even if you had previously lost all desire.

I'm not too surprised by Desiree's success. As your FAT programs get turned off through visualization, you'll naturally have more energy to be active. Remember, one of the chemical changes that takes place when you're leptin resistant is that the brain sends fewer messages to the thyroid to produce thyroid hormones. This slows your metabolism and makes you feel tired and lethargic. That's an intentional act on the part of the body to conserve calories. When your FAT programs are on, just the thought of exercise is exhausting. When I was overweight, walking up a flight of stairs seemed daunting.

However, as your chemistry changes, your thyroid speeds up and you have much more energy. Suddenly, the idea of being physically active is appealing. You'll be drawn to activities that you loved as a child or that you are intrigued by as an adult.

VISUALIZATION FOR RECONNECTING WITH THE JOY OF MOVEMENT

Many of the people I speak with tell me how much they hate exercise. They groan if I even bring it up. But when we were children, we ran, we jumped, we chased balls, and we chased each other, without ever realizing we were "exercising." Activity has gotten a bad rap because we've been told we must do it. And it has been stripped of its pleasure by so-called experts who want us do hours of mindless, repetitive, boring aerobic exercise.

You can recapture the joy you experienced as a child by visualizing an activity you once loved to do:

> Once you're in SMART Mode (see pages 20–21), picture yourself in your ideal body, toned and firm and strong and fast and lean. Feel the wind in your hair as you're running to get the ball. Feel the sun on your shoulders, hear the ocean and birds, smell the salt air; use all your senses to really be in the scene, loving the feeling of being active and enjoying your fit, energetic body.

Try this at night before you go to bed or first thing in the morning—especially on days when you actually intend to be active. By visualizing the inherent fun in the activity of your choice, you'll begin changing the dysfunctional belief that you don't like movement and you'll be creating and reinforcing powerful neural connections and associating the physical with fun, love, and joy.

IMPROVING YOUR RESULTS

Visualization doesn't just help you find the joy in movement so you move more; it actually has the power to boost the quality and results of the exercise you are doing. Many professional athletes rely on visualization to reach and then remain at the top of their game. Golfing great Jack Nicklaus and gold-medal Olympic gymnast Mary Lou Retton both credit their success to visualization. Premier League soccer forward Didier Drogba visualizes his strikes in advance: "I actually think about the way I am going to score my goal," he says. "When you get it in your head that you are going to score a certain kind of goal, it happens."[1]

Researchers have found that nerve receptors in your muscles actually fire when you visualize activity. In 2013, researchers at the University of Texas asked college students to imagine lifting a heavy weight with their right arms for a few minutes, five days a week. When the researchers monitored brain waves and muscle contractions, they found that the students' brains were sending nerve impulses to muscles as if they were actually working their arms. After six weeks, the researchers measured the students' right arm strength: they were 11 percent stronger, and the students hadn't hefted a single dumbbell.[2]

Even when visualization is pitted against actual gym workouts, it fares well. Exercise psychologist Guang Yue at the Cleveland Clinic in Ohio compared people who exercised at a gym with people who only visualized doing similar workouts. After three months, Yue discovered that the visualizers had increased their muscle strength by almost half as much (13 percent) as the gym-goers (30 percent).[3] Again, the visualizers hadn't lifted a *single weight.*

VISUALIZE A NEW WAY TO BE ACTIVE

At the Gabriel Method, we avoid the word *workout* because it implies that we're doing work to our outer body only—the stereotypical calorie-burning routine—which is ultimately pointless and rarely effective. Instead, I like to talk about "work-ins," where we use specific types of exercise combined with visualization to create an internal shift in our biochemistry. Exercise done right shouldn't feel like work. It should feel like play, and the changes that happen will be cumulative over time, creating a positive spiral of fitness in your life.

I came to realize from my own experience that activity should be fun. I couldn't spend hours on treadmills or lifting weights. The repetition was just too boring; I wasn't having fun. I suspect you may be like me in this. Don't blame yourself if you dread going to the gym and trudging on a stair stepper. The evidence is piling up that steady-paced aerobic workouts are not only unhelpful; *they may actually interfere with your weight loss.* They can lead to a phenomenon known as "overtraining," which creates a type of chronic stress in the body that can actually activate your FAT programs, just like so many other low-level chronic stresses. When it comes to boosting fitness and shedding pounds, quick bursts of activity—the kind you get when playing tennis or basketball, riding a bike up and down hills, or chasing and wrestling with your kids—can't be beat.

Based on countless studies, health experts at the U.S. Department of Health and Human Services and the American College of Sports Medicine now recommend against relying solely on steady-paced aerobic exercise to help you lose weight.[4]

There is a much better way to use exercise for weight loss. Shorter, more intense bursts of exercise activate your inside-out weight loss mechanisms, and research is very clear about this. Exercise scientists at McMaster University in Canada asked volunteers to alternate minute-long bouts of fast pedaling on a stationary bike with short periods of rest for 20 minutes. After doing this three times a week for two weeks, the volunteers had gained as much endurance as people who had spun the pedals at a moderate pace for an hour a day, five days a week.[5] You'll shed more fat this way, too. Canadian researchers found that just two weeks of interval training (this is the term for short-burst, high-intensity exercise) enabled women to burn *36 percent more fat.*[6] And a study from the United Kingdom revealed that just four to six 30-second sprints on a stationary bike boosted levels of human growth hormone *530 percent.*[7] Human growth hormone builds muscle and burns fat.

If you're wondering whether this really leads to weight loss, the answer is yes: Australian researchers found that the women doing only 20 minutes of intervals lost almost six pounds on average without dieting, while women cycling at a moderate pace for 40 minutes actually *gained* weight.[8]

Although the studies on interval training required people to perform regimented timed bouts of sprinting and active rest, you don't have to use a stopwatch and a heart-rate monitor to achieve these results. You can get the same effect by pursuing the activities you love. Most games have natural fast-paced and slow-paced rhythms. Bicycling on roads or hiking on trails requires intense effort going uphill and provide a chance to catch your breath when going downhill and on the flats. Most ball sports involve fast bursts, then rest, so do dancing, skiing, playing chase in the park with kids, or water sports like surfing, kayaking, kite surfing, and polo. In fact, most sports that are designed to be fun follow this pattern. So for me, when it comes to fitness, fun is really where it's at.

THE GET-THIN-OR-GET-EATEN ADAPTATION

There's another reason the short-burst approach to exercise is so effective. Along with the FAT programs that *force* you to gain weight to help you endure long winters, you also have other survival programs in your brain that *force* you to lose weight—also for survival reasons. Basically, it's a survival program that evolved to protect you from predators. I call it the "get-thin-or-get-eaten" adaptation.

If you were living outdoors thousands of years ago and a predator like a bear or tiger leaped out, you wouldn't have been able to survive by going for a 40-minute power walk. You would need a full-out, life-or-death sprint. At that moment, you'd get a surge of adrenaline, and your muscles would demand more energy *now*. Together, this would signal to your survival brain that you're living in an environment where you need to be lean, and it would respond by activating your get-thin-or-get-eaten adaptation. Your sensitivity to leptin would increase—and research demonstrates that short-burst exercise does in fact raise your leptin sensitivity—which in turn boosts your ability to burn fat and lose weight.

I experienced this in a very real way when I was about three-quarters through my weight loss journey. I was biking this beautiful route that followed winding, hilly dirt roads through vineyards. As I pedaled, I was musing about what might help take my progress to the next level. Suddenly, a dog came out of nowhere and started chasing me. I had to sprint for a mile or so with this beast barking and snapping a millimeter from my Achilles tendon.

I managed to escape without injury, but it took a while for my heart and breathing to return to normal. Then, over the next couple of weeks, I noticed a big change: without doing anything different, I began dropping weight like crazy!

My brush with the dog had activated my get-thin-or-get-eaten adaptation, and my survival brain took over. Although I wasn't doing anything differently, I wasn't as hungry and the weight was falling off. I began shedding pounds more rapidly because my body had made a primal association between being fast and thin and surviving.

Once I realized what had happened, I began to repeat the scenario that had given me such positive results. Whenever I got to that same place on my bike ride, I would stand and sprint while *imagining* that dog was chasing me. (I'm happy to say, I never saw the actual dog again.) The simulation worked as well as the real thing—my weight loss accelerated. In this way I learned to use visualization to activate the get-thin-or-get-eaten adaptation.

USE VISUALIZATION TO TRIGGER THE GET-THIN-OR-GET-EATEN ADAPTATION

To get these effects for yourself, you don't have to look for a dog to chase you. If you're going for a walk or a bike ride, begin at a leisurely pace. Then, every once in a while, go as fast as you possibly can for 10 or 20 seconds while imagining that you're being chased by something—like I did after my initial experience. Your survival brain doesn't know the difference between real and imagined experiences. By planting the idea that you're being chased, you're convincing your survival brain that you're *actually being chased by a predator,* and this activates the get-thin-or-get-eaten adaptation. If imagining a predator chasing you is too uncomfortable, just imagine you're being chased by a friend but that you are deter-mined to beat him at all costs. You'll still get great results.

After a while of doing the visualization of being chased while I was biking, I decided to try an experiment. I took my visualization one step further and just *imagined* that I was riding my bike and that the dog was chasing me, without actually exercising at all. Remarkably, that worked, too! I went through a period of several weeks where I did no exercise at all. But as I was going to sleep at night, I visualized the scene of biking really hard with my trusty canine companion snapping at my heels. I imagined that I was in the best shape of my life and sprinting at a blinding pace. I saw myself easily outpacing the dog and even smiling because I was moving so fast and it was so easy to escape. During those sever-al weeks of using only visualization, my fitness continued to im-prove, just as it did for the exercisers in the visualization studies.

In other words, because the survival brain can't differentiate between a real and imagined experience, you can simply picture yourself sprinting and your chemistry will change as if you were actually being active.

You may be thinking, isn't that stress, being chased by a dog? Isn't stress bad for you? The answer is yes and no. From a weight loss perspective, it depends on what the stress is, how your body interprets the stress, and, most important, how your body *adapts* to the stress.

Our bodies are brilliantly designed to adapt to any stress in our environment. If the stress is a famine, the body turns on the FAT programs, making you insatiably hungry so you'll gain more weight. Having extra weight on your body during times of famine is less stressful; the fat can help keep you alive. But if you're being chased by a tiger—a different kind of stress—the brain will adapt by making you as thin and fit as possible to help you survive.

As a result, imagining you're being chased can be an extremely powerful visualization technique. See yourself easily outrunning your pursuer and leaving the beast far behind you. Keep a smile on your face in the visualization. See your body as being strong and fast as the wind, so fast that nothing could ever catch you.

And remember, if the predator chase is too much, too intense, you can always imagine being chased by a friend. These images will have the same effect of communicating to your survival brain that you need to be thin.

One last note: if you're visualizing *while* exercising, remember that you shouldn't do it daily. Overtraining, as I mentioned, can actually turn on your FAT programs. With a few sessions of activity a week combined with daily visualizations, you'll tap into this powerful survival adaptation by convincing your body to *want* to be thin.

For a full guided get-thin-or-get-eaten visualization, called Activate the "Get Thin" Programs with Movement, please see pages 175–176.

Visualization can help us reconnect with our bodies, but it also helps with something else that's essential for weight loss, as we'll talk about in the next chapter. It's so essential that many researchers believe it's the most crucial ingredient to health, happiness, and sustainable fitness: sleep.

CHAPTER 9

SLEEP YOUR WAY TO SLENDERNESS

W̲e tend to take sleep for granted. Hit the sack, get as many hours as a hectic schedule allows, and then rise to a blaring alarm clock. A shower, coffee, and a busy workday help keep us on our feet and stumbling through our day, even if we're weighed down by fatigue with every step.

Sleep is so underrated that we allow almost anything to get in the way of a solid eight hours. Our modern life has us blinking under bright artificial lights, idling the evenings away on the Internet, and watching late-night television programs. According to international surveys, most residents of developed countries sleep between five and six hours nightly.

The body and brain need more. The results of poor, minimal sleep show up in the increased risks of heart disease, type 2 diabetes, and, of course, weight gain. You may be relieved to hear that an incredibly effective weight loss strategy is to simply sleep better—and more—than you currently do. Even better, taking time for your evening visualization can go a long way to ensuring that you do sleep well. But first you have to rule out an insidious robber of rest that plagues overweight people.

THE SLEEP THIEF

When someone comes to me looking to lose at least 75 pounds, the first thing I ask them is whether they've been checked for sleep apnea. I battled this devastating condition myself, and I would never have been able to lose so much weight without getting treatment.

Someone with sleep apnea continually and repeatedly stops breathing during sleep. (*Apnea* is a Greek word that literally means "without breath.") The condition is characterized by window-rattling snores, long gaps in breathing, and gasping as the sufferer struggles for air. The reason for these symptoms is that airways actually collapse during sleep; sufferers can go a minute or longer without breathing. Unfortunately, you wouldn't realize you have it because people with sleep apnea don't fully wake up during an episode. However, they never reach deep sleep, either, and as a result they're always sleep deprived.

For a long time, sleep specialists thought that sleep apnea was purely a result of weight gain—that being overweight put a person at risk for sleep apnea. That's because fatty deposits gather in the neck, causing the airways to collapse during sleep. But more recently, researchers have discovered that sleep apnea can actually *cause* weight gain, too—it goes both ways! In 2011, sleep scientists at the University of Arizona reported results from a long-term sleep apnea study. The researchers tracked 3,001 men and women who fell into one of three categories: they had no symptoms of sleep apnea, intermittent symptoms, or severe apnea. After five years, the researchers found that patients with the most severe cases had gained twice as much weight as those with few symptoms.[1]

Sleep apnea triggers weight gain because it activates your FAT programs. Long gaps in breathing every night put the body under chronic stress. As research clearly shows, chronic stress causes the release of cortisol and other stress hormones that signal to your brain that it's time to hoard fat and slow down metabolism. The stress spills over into your waking hours, as well, because anyone with sleep apnea understandably lacks energy as they go through their day. Battling low energy on a daily basis causes junk food cravings and further fuels FAT programs.

A few years ago, a guy named Alan called me. He lived in Melbourne and wanted to talk to me about losing weight. He went on about his physical trainers, his diet, and how many calories he eats on good days and bad days. But the whole time Alan was talking I could hear his heavy, labored breathing over the phone. I immediately suspected that he might have sleep apnea, and I asked if he had been to see a sleep specialist.

At first Alan was resistant. "I sleep okay," he said, and kept talking about his exercise and food habits. I finally stopped him and said, "I don't want to talk about those details yet. First, you need to get checked for sleep apnea." We've been so conditioned to believe that weight gain is a result of eating too much or moving too little that we often fail to see huge problems with our health that are directly related to the weight. I finally convinced Alan that before he did anything else to try and lose weight, he needed to see a specialist.

Four months went by before I heard from Alan again. Then, out of the blue, he called to tell me some happy news: he had lost 88 pounds in four months. And he hadn't spent any extra time obsessing over his fitness plan or his diet. All he had done was get treatment for his sleep apnea, and the weight had just fallen off.

I knew that Alan would begin to lose weight after managing his sleep apnea because that's what happened to me. I had a world-class case of sleep apnea. My wife used to sleep with earplugs, and she had spare earplugs for guests when they visited. I remember one time I was on a long flight sitting at the back of the plane. I dozed off for a bit. When I opened my eyes, every single person on the plane as far as I could see was peering over the back of their seats at me. Rows and rows and rows, little kids, parents, elderly folks—they had all turned around and were staring at me because of my snoring.

Getting a sleep apnea diagnosis means that you may have to spend the night in a sleep laboratory hooked up to electrodes that track your breathing and brain waves. That may sound like a hassle, but when you consider all the crazy things we try in the effort to lose weight, a night in a sleep laboratory is actually very reasonable and cost-effective. And, unlike diets, getting checked for sleep apnea addresses a real issue rather than offering a Band-Aid approach.

My sleep apnea was revealed when I was at a sleep laboratory. Although I was supposed to spend the entire night, within two hours the sleep technicians woke me up to tell me I definitely had sleep apnea; in fact, I had one of the worst cases they had ever seen. Pretty much the whole time I was gasping for air.

The sleep technicians put me on a CPAP (continuous positive airway pressure) machine, a mask that you wear that blows air into your nose and mouth. The air pressure prevents the airways from collapsing. Once the technicians got the pressure to the right level, I got my first good night's sleep in years. When I woke up, my mind was clear and calm. For the first time in years, I actually had dreams. I was relaxed, my stress levels went down, and my energy and clarity increased.

Depending on how serious your sleep apnea is, you might be able to manage it with nasal decongestants, sleeping on your side, or wearing a specially designed mouthpiece that puts the jaw in a position that helps keep airways open. Some people resort to surgery. Regardless of the route you take, managing sleep apnea has to be a priority.

WHY YOU NEED TO SLEEP MORE

Even if you don't have sleep apnea, there's a good chance you're not getting enough shut-eye. In 2004, Stanford scientists tracked the sleep patterns of 1,000 people in Wisconsin and found that the less sleep someone got, the heavier they were. And there was a tipping point: sleeping less than six hours a night was significantly linked to obesity.[2]

Researchers at the University of Chicago, led by Eve Van Cauter, a sleep specialist, asked a group of healthy men to sleep for only four hours a night for two nights. Afterward, Van Cauter ran blood tests and tracked the men's eating. She found that the men ate 24 percent more calories mostly in the form of sugary and fatty foods. The blood tests revealed dramatic changes in the men's hormones: levels of the hunger hormone ghrelin climbed, while levels of leptin—which suppresses appetite—fell.[3]

In 2010, researchers at the University of Chicago found that people who are trying to lose weight will lose *twice as much fat* when they get a full night's sleep.[4] This study also revealed that sleeping less than six hours a night raises levels of ghrelin, triggering hunger and slowing metabolism. It also decreases sensitivity to leptin and insulin.

When you fail to get enough sleep, your brain can spur you to make poor choices the following day. A Harvard study published in the journal *Sleep* around the same time found sleep-deprived teens favored fatty food and snacks compared with teens who got a solid eight hours. In fact, for each hour increase of sleep (up to eight), the odds that a teen would consume extra junk calories declined 21 percent.[5]

Living life sleep deprived leads to more than weight gain. A ten-year study of more than 71,000 women found that those who slept five hours or less on a typical night were up to 45 percent more likely to suffer heart attacks than women who slept eight hours.[6] Japanese scientists tracked the sleep habits of 1,255 people with high blood pressure for nearly two years. They found that those who slept fewer than 7.5 hours per night, on average, increased their risk of heart attack or stroke by 68 percent.[7]

Sleep supports the health of your entire body. Specialists at the University of Pittsburgh School of Medicine have found that a number of bodily systems suffer when we don't sleep enough: the heart, lungs, and kidneys don't function properly, immunity to infection weakens, the risk of depression and other mood disorders rise, and appetite soars while metabolism slows down.[8] How can poor sleep cause so much harm? Sleep is how your body recharges its batteries. The brain slides into restorative wave patterns that heal the body and prepare it for the challenges ahead. Memories are formed, learning is made concrete, and bodily functions are reenergized. As you fall asleep, your brain passes through an alpha wave state, the same brain wave state we elicit through visualization. Once you're asleep, you'll then go much deeper into the theta and delta states associated with memory, emotions, and rejuvenation.

But when you deprive your body of these brain states, you're putting your body under constant chronic stress, and the results can be seen in the studies above. Your body releases the stress hormone cortisol, which activates your FAT programs, and your body begins going into chronic fat storage mode.

Weight troubles accelerate exponentially should you develop sleep apnea. Now you're waking several times a night, you almost never reach a state of deep, restorative sleep, and cortisol levels go up even further. You're in a vicious cycle where the body responds by further decreasing sensitivity to leptin, slowing your metabolism, and putting you on a ravenous hunt for energy in the form of calories.

GET YOUR ZZZS BACK

Once you've been checked for sleep apnea and successfully treated, there's another option for making sure your sleep is restful, deep, and restorative: visualization. When Vicki first began the evening visualizations with the Gabriel Method, she hadn't slept well for years. Her insomnia took the form of waking in the middle of the night and being unable to fall back asleep. This changed with her first visualization: "Once I started doing the bedtime meditation, I slept through the night seven nights in a row!" she says. "This is huge. I'm convinced it's the visualization."

There's no question that it's the mind-body relaxation technique of visualization that's helping. Researchers have used visualization and similar mind-body techniques like meditation and kriya yoga—which is a form of guided-imagery meditation similar to SMART Mode—to help people sleep better. When researchers at Northwestern University compared insomniacs who were taught kriya yoga with those who were given basic information on how to sleep better, after two months the researchers found that the yoga group fell asleep faster, slept longer, and spent more time in deep sleep.[9]

Just how powerful can guided-imagery meditation—a form of visualization—be in helping people reach sound sleep? Researchers at the University of Minnesota tested regular guided-imagery-based meditation against a top-selling prescription sleep drug. The researchers recruited 30 insomniacs. Half of the patients began practicing daily guided imagery; the rest were given a prescription for the sleep drug Lunesta. After two months, the people who used guided-imagery meditation were sleeping much better than they were at the beginning of the study. What's more, they were sleeping as soundly as the people taking the sleep drug. After another three months, the researchers checked in with the volunteers and found that the guided-imagery group was actually doing better than the medication group.[10]

The University of Minnesota researchers also reported that the guided-imagery participants were much happier with their treatment than the group taking pills was; they reported an overall improvement in their quality of life.[11]

Taking time for an evening visualization will improve your sleep almost immediately. Linda found that she began falling asleep faster after just two days of doing the evening visualization. "I started sleeping more peacefully than I could believe possible," she says. "And the next day, my craving for sweets was almost gone."

Nearly any type of visualization practice will be immediately helpful, but one of the reasons the Gabriel Method visualizations are so powerful is that we use a "frequency-following" pattern in the background. Frequency-following means that the music has a beat that encourages your brain to cycle at the same frequency as the music. As the visualization progresses, that cycle slows. Your brain waves will start to follow this pattern. By the end of the visualization, you will drift deeper and deeper into sleep. Some people worry that they're falling asleep during the visualization, but they shouldn't. It's designed to help you sleep, and your subconscious will still be just as receptive to the positive suggestions as when you are awake.

GABRIELIZE YOUR SLEEP HABITS AND BEDROOM

If you set a regular bedtime routine, you'll train your body to slow down and have an easier time falling asleep. I have a little ritual that I do sometimes: I take a hot bath or shower in which I make the water progressively warmer as I become accustomed to the temperature. After I get out, I do a gentle stretch or two, such as a simple hamstring stretch or the child's pose in yoga in which I get on my knees, forehead touching the ground, and stretch my hands out in front of me for a minute or two.

Then I get into bed, breathe slowly and deeply, and start my visualization.

You'll soon find that sleeping better will give you more energy and clarity, reduce sugar cravings, and accelerate weight loss.

Remember, you can download our evening visualization for free at www.TheGabrielMethod.com/freecd.

CHAPTER 10

OVERCOME FOOD CRAVINGS AND ADDICTIONS

Cravings are all anyone ever wants to talk about when they are on a diet or weight loss program. I personally place little emphasis on resisting cravings, because I know that the cravings are always a symptom, never the cause of the problem. For example, if you're craving potato chips, it can mean that your body actually needs more healthy fats and trace minerals. Sugar cravings typically mean that you're insulin resistant and have lost the ability to regulate your blood sugar properly. You can become insulin resistant from being nutritionally starved or from chronic stress.

Learning how to manage your stress and nourish your body properly will go a long way toward making those cravings disappear. I've seen it happen thousands of times: after beginning to work with visualization, clients say, "I just don't crave sweets anymore." It makes perfect sense. When you take an inside-out approach to weight loss, you're changing your body on a cellular and chemical level, so the cravings are being eliminated from their source.

If you've already started practicing daily visualizations, you may find your attraction to junk food and sweets diminishing on its own. As your FAT programs begin to shut down, high-calorie, high-fat foods begin to seem less appealing. Following the inside-out approach to weight loss naturally triggers a desire for healthier foods. You won't crave those extreme flavor blasts of tooth-aching sweetness and mouth-puckering saltiness. Once your brain accepts that it's time to get thinner, you'll naturally crave high-nutrient, sensible foods like fresh produce, nuts and seeds, sprouted beans—foods that at one point you may have thought you could never crave will suddenly seem very appealing.

The reason you'll be drawn to healthier food is that your body is trying to lose weight. It wants to be thinner, and as your cells become more sensitive to leptin and insulin, you'll feel full sooner. Your urges will automatically steer you toward healthier foods—the ones that give you the highest-quality bang for your nutritional buck.

However, we all have weaknesses, and it just so happens that visualization is extremely effective for killing junk food cravings and food addictions. So if you don't want to wait for the inside-out approach to naturally dissolve your junk food cravings, you can use specific visualization techniques to accelerate the process.

At the moment you might feel that certain foods "have power" over you. You might lose control at the sight of chocolate cake. Other people might be brought to their knees by a pint of cookie-dough ice cream. Maybe salty snacks are your weakness, with BBQ potato chips and french fries singing a constant siren song in the back of your mind. Whatever your nutritional Achilles' heel might be, visualization can help bring it under control.

HOW VISUALIZATION STIFLES CRAVINGS

My weakness as a young teenager was sugar. While I wasn't heavy yet—not like I was later, when I was working on Wall Street—I was a pudgy kid, and I was particularly attracted to sugar. I'd ladle it onto my breakfast cereal, sprinkle it on waffles, and even sneak it out of the bowl by the spoonful.

About the time I was realizing that I needed to do something about my sugar habit, my aunt came to visit my family in Philadelphia. I was serving her some coffee, and I asked her how much sugar she wanted. She said, "I don't take sugar." I was surprised. Nearly every adult I knew put sugar in their coffee. (A "regular coffee" in that part of the world means you want it with cream and sugar.)

I had to ask my aunt again, "You don't have sugar in your coffee?" She replied that she didn't eat sugar at all, period. I was stunned. How could she never eat sugar? The concept seemed so foreign to me. But I began to wonder, could I give up sugar? I asked my aunt how she had accomplished this incredible feat, and she explained that she had done it through visualization. A light went on for me, because I was able to control my migraines with the same method. Could visualization actually help me conquer my sugar cravings, as well?

My aunt let me in on the secret of how she beat her sugar cravings. During visualization, while in a deep meditative state, she imagined that sugar granules were actually little pieces of ground glass. I tried it immediately. I began my visualization by slowly calming my mind and sliding down into a suggestive mental state; then I pictured what would happen if I put these sugar granules—which were ground glass—in my mouth. They were tasteless. Worse, they would cut up my mouth and destroy my insides. I was repulsed.

After a few days of doing this visualization, I didn't want sweets at all. The effect was so strong that I didn't eat sugar for almost 12 years. I couldn't even look at a donut. If I walked by a bakery, I'd get nauseous. Just like that, the craving was gone. I had artificially created an aversion that—to my brain—seemed very real.

This approach has worked for countless Gabriel Method participants. Nicole had struggled with her cravings for decades when she finally discovered visualization. Once she forged a connection between chocolate—her weakness—and stinky, foul mud, her desire soon abated. "I was amazed that my cravings disappeared in just two weeks."

Meredith began getting results even faster. "After just three days, my cravings are changing," she said. "I don't want sugar anymore, and that's amazing for me."

In 2005, researchers at Flinders University in Adelaide, Australia, recruited 130 students and asked them to imagine eating a favorite food. The researchers really put the students through their paces by making them remember in detail every aspect of the food. If the student was imagining sitting down to a steak, he would picture the sizzle, the texture, the smell, and, of course, the taste. As the students recalled their indulgence, they rated what made them most crave the food: Was it the taste? The smell? Or was it the mental image of the food that triggered their desire? When the researchers went over the students' responses, they found that mental images were by far the most powerful driver of cravings. A vivid mental picture increased the intensity of desire much more than memories of taste or smell did.[1]

The Australian researchers concluded that the most effective way to battle unwanted food cravings would be to interfere with that compelling mental image. They decided to try distracting volunteers to lessen cravings and help them avoid obsessing over a food. In a subsequent study, the researchers had 50 women perform distracting tasks while they pictured the foods that they craved. The women would look at abstract images, for example, or tap an imaginary line in front of their faces with their fingers to avoid focusing on the food.

The distractions worked well: the women reported that temptation was less of an issue when they used these techniques.[2] However, the distractions only served to tone down the effect of the image, not eliminate it—or better yet—render it undesirable. That's where visualization comes in.

Consider this for a moment. If you tell yourself that chocolate cake is bad, and that you shouldn't eat it, what happens? All you can do is picture that chocolate cake and you start salivating. As the Australian researchers found, picturing the cake is the single worst thing you can do if you're trying to resist temptation. The image of that cake makes you want it so much more.

Trying to rely on willpower to resist your cravings will only make the food that much more desirable. That's where the term *forbidden fruit* originates. You just end up magnetizing your attraction and desire for the very food you're trying to avoid. Trying to tell your brain to ignore it won't work for long. After all, your survival brain doesn't respond to verbal commands. You need images to get through to it. And if you choose the right images, not only can you convince your survival brain that the food is something to avoid, but you'll actually be repulsed by the very food that once drove you crazy.

HOW VISUALIZATION STOPS ADDICTION

You can see how visualization grants you mastery over your cravings. But what about addictions? As a young teen, I also started smoking. But I was also an athlete. I played soccer and I was a ski racer. I began to see that smoking and sports were incompatible. Again, I thought I would try visualization. It had worked for my sugar cravings, after all. What if I could create a negative connection with tobacco that would eliminate my desire for cigarettes?

It actually turns out that food and drug cravings are not so different, as researchers at the Monell Chemical Senses Center in Philadelphia discovered. In 2004, they asked volunteers to imagine their favorite foods—the foods they most often craved—while undergoing an MRI of the brain. The researchers discovered that picturing the food activated the same brain structures that light up when addicted drug users imagine their vices.[3] In fact, food and drug addictions are so similar that one research report recently found that cocaine and heroin are less addictive than Oreo cookies.[4]

But it turns out that visualization is an effective treatment for both. In a research report titled "A Study of Visualization and Addiction Treatment," psychologist Kathryn Kominars, at Florida International University in Miami, tested visualization with 76 addicts over eight months. Kominars compared visualization with typical psychological education and counseling for addiction. She found that visualization could help addicts beat their problems and deal with the temptation as well—and in some cases better— than the standard treatment.[5]

That's how I ended up kicking my cigarette addiction. After getting into my visualization, I pictured the tar and nicotine in tobacco as the same thing as the hot tar road crews use to repair asphalt. I imagined that the second I brought a cigarette to my mouth, it was full of that hot, stinky tar. If I inhaled it, I would be drawing that greasy tar deep into my lungs. The image was so repulsive that I was able to stop smoking the next day. I kept up the visualization for a few more weeks, and that was the end of my smoking habit.

From then on, if I touched a cigarette I would immediately get that association. If you ever question the power of these associations, just imagine taking a bite out of a sandwich and then noticing there are maggots crawling inside. You would immediately spit it out, and whatever was in that sandwich—turkey, ham, bologna—you would be so repulsed by it that it might take years before you'd feel comfortable eating that meat again. This actually happened to a friend of mine. She loved oysters in a tin and ate them frequently. But several years ago, she got a bad batch and became violently ill. To this day she can't even look at oysters without getting an upset stomach.

So you can try imagining sugar as ground glass, bread full of maggots, or chocolate as mud. Be creative; the more repulsive the association, the more effective. I know a man who, as a child, ate a sandwich that someone had spit in without telling him. Once he found out, he couldn't eat another sandwich for 30 years! From one extremely unpleasant association, he's spent his entire adult life not eating bread. You can use the power of your mind in this way to create negative associations to problematic foods and addictions.

VISUALIZATION TO OVERCOME CRAVINGS AND FOOD ADDICTIONS

If you're looking to beat a craving or tame an addiction, try the visualization below and come up with a truly disgusting image that you can associate with your problem. You'll be surprised how fast you will be able to make dramatic changes.

While in SMART mode (see pages 20–21), imagine yourself about to eat the specific food you'd like to avoid. After you've taken a bite of the food, look at it and notice what's different. Maybe it's really mud and not chocolate; maybe there are maggots crawling around in it. Quickly spit out the mouthful and throw the food on the ground.

Feel every cell of your body saying at the same time, "This food is disgusting; it's repulsive."

Now imagine that you're walking past a bakery or restaurant where you see this specific food and feel your stomach start to tighten and your body contract, and feel how every cell of your body is repulsed by the sight and smell of the food. See yourself quickly walking past the store in disgust.

Later, imagine you're craving healthy, live, vibrant, nutritious foods. See yourself eating them and loving them. Feel every cell of your body delight at the taste and the nourishment you're getting. See yourself getting fitter and healthier and more vibrant as the days go by and as you're craving only real, live, healthy, nourishing foods. And see the weight effortlessly melting off your body.

Again this type of visualization doesn't actually address the root causes of a problem. You may very well find that you won't need this method because the other inside-out work you are doing will take care of your cravings or addictions. But this approach can be useful if you want to accelerate the changes you're making or if you have a serious addiction that you're battling to a food or drug. There's no better way to kick a habit than being repulsed by the substance.

CHAPTER 11

SEVEN STEPS TO A PERFECT VISUALIZATION

W e've been discussing visualization in connection with nearly every aspect of your physical and mental health, from sleep to exercise to cravings, habits, beliefs, stress reduction, trauma relief, and even genetics. Now it's time to learn exactly how to practice visualization—and, more important, how to create your own perfect visualization. With the information you learn in this chapter, you'll be able to tap into this extremely powerful technique and start reaping the benefits quickly. You'll only need about five or ten minutes to walk yourself through this process. I also have three guided visualizations that you can listen to that will help you learn. Find these at www.TheGabrielMethod.com /visualization-bonus.

PROPER SITTING POSTURE

Before we get started, let's talk about the best way to sit for visualization. For a morning or daytime visualization, sit in a chair that has your hips slightly higher than your knees when your feet are planted flat on the floor. Sit up straight on the edge of the chair. If possible, your back shouldn't be touching the chairback or a cushion. If that isn't comfortable for you, rest your back on the chair or pillow. Clasp your hands together comfortably in your lap, and tuck your chin slightly in to help straighten the length of your spine. Your goal is to keep your spine straight throughout your visualization.

:an, breathe only through your nose and keep your
:d, jaw relaxed, and your tongue lightly touching the
mouth. This completes an energy circuit according to
Chinese traditional medicine, and it's something we'll talk about
more in Chapter 13.

Just remember that your overall goal with your posture is to be
comfortable. If any of these things make you uncomfortable, don't
do them. If you need to open your mouth to breathe easily, that's
totally fine. Again, if you're more comfortable with your back supported, slide back on your seat. For me to be comfortable, I put a
pillow in my lap to rest my hands on so they're not too low. This
helps me keep my back straight with less effort.

For the evening visualization, you'll be laying down because
the goal is to relax into sleep. For all other visualizations, sitting is
the ideal position.

Try to breathe through your belly and not your chest. Just let
your belly expand when you inhale and contract when you ex-
hale. Picture a circle of light like a pinwheel circling around your
navel. Each time you breathe, imagine the air entering and es-
caping through your navel, and it spins the pinwheel. When you
breathe in, it spins faster and then slows; when you breathe out,
it spins again. Picturing the pinwheel will keep your mind and
energy focused inside your body.

Now, here are seven simple steps to help you create the
perfect visualization.

STEP 1: GET INTO SMART MODE

As with all my visualizations, the first thing is to get your
mind into the more powerful, highly programmable state of
SMART Mode. You'll slow your brain waves down to the alpha and
theta states as we discussed earlier. These wavelengths indicate
your mind is in a creative state; unlike the beta state, which is
where your brain is as you're going about your usual business.
SMART Mode is the energy and the driving force behind your
visualization—it's the reason visualizing works.

There are several ways to get into SMART Mode, in addition to the one you learned back in Chapter 2. It's really about bringing your awareness into your body and being in the present moment. You can get there by stretching, meditating, journaling, painting, walking in nature, taking a hot bath, making love (who said it can't be fun!), exercising, or doing yoga, tai chi, or qigong. You can also listen to frequency-following music, like the music on our website. As we talked about, the music has a frequency built into it that is similar to the alpha and theta state, and your brain will entrain with that frequency. Baroque music also typically has patterns similar to the alpha state.

Hypnotherapists get patients into SMART Mode through suggestion. They guide their patients systematically through the body. Starting with the feet, for example, and suggesting that each part of the body relax and let go. You can try this yourself. Imagine relaxing your toes, then heels, then ankles, calves, knees, thighs, and so on, until you've reached your scalp. As you progress through the body relaxing all the muscles and joints, your brain calms down and your awareness shifts to your physical being.

The most natural way to reach this state is through visualization. There are many ways you can use visualization to get into SMART Mode. All you need is to find imagery that relaxes you simply and relatively quickly.

I like to use the imagery of white light spreading through the body. There are numerous health benefits associated with imagining white light energizing your body, and we'll talk about these benefits in the next chapter. I have two simple visualizations that use white light to help relax your body. One is called the "spinning the spine" technique (see the next page) and the other is the "ocean of energy" visualization you learned in Chapter 2. You can use whichever one speaks most to you. Both take just a few minutes and help you easily transition into the next steps of your visualization.

(Note: This is an actual transcript of a live, guided visualization. The causal language style and occasional redundant statements are intentional as they help you get into the ideal meditative state.)

> Imagine a glowing ball of white light, about the size of a golf ball, starting at your navel, then going down to the base of the spine and spinning around each vertebra, one at a time. You have 24 vertebrae in your spine. Don't worry about exactly where each vertebra is, just imagine the ball of light spinning around the base of your spine a few times and then going up one notch at a time, 24 times. After you've gone up about five notches, you should imagine the ball of light to be around the middle of your stomach, then after about 12 to 14 vertebrae, behind your heart. When it gets to 17, you're in your neck, and when you get to 24 you're at the base of the skull. Then imagine the ball of light going into your head, then your face, front of your neck, your heart, and then again into your stomach. By the time the ball gets back to your stomach, you should be in SMART Mode. Now imagine the ball of light expanding to cover every part of your body, so that every cell is glowing with white light.

Don't worry if you can't "see" these things happening; just imagine it, pretend it, and "feel" it any way that you can. It's the process that's important here, because doing the process of practicing this imagery puts you in the ideal brain wave state.

Once again, please see Chapter 2 or Appendix B for the ocean of light visualization for getting into SMART Mode. That happens to be the one I use most frequently at the moment as I find it's slightly faster and simpler.

STEP 2: MAKE AFFIRMATIONS

Now that you're aware of every cell of your body and imagining every cell of your body glowing with white light, it's a perfect time to start communicating with your cells. You can use an affirmation to make any desired change you'd like, whether it's to change a habit, belief, or food choice; break an addiction; or anything else. Just make sure that the words you use in your affirmation focus on the positive and take place in the present (not future) tense. So, for example, you can say, "Weight loss is easy," rather than "Soon weight loss won't be hard for me."

Once you have your affirmation, picture every cell of your body repeating it: *Weight loss is easy. I love myself. I forgive myself. I crave real, live, vibrant foods. I feel safe, strong, and protected. Life is safe. I am safe. I am loved. Abundance easily and effortlessly flows to me.* Remember, this can focus on any change you'd like to create in your life. I recommend that you repeat these affirmations for a minute or two, imagining that every cell in your body is repeating the words in unison.

STEP 3: MELT THE WEIGHT OFF

After you finish your affirmations, imagine that any excess weight you have on your body has become a white light and is getting sucked into the center of your navel. You can imagine that the pinwheel we talked about in step 1 has become a vortex of spinning light in your navel or a whirlpool that is sucking excess fat into it. Picture the excess fat on your body as something that is no longer physical, but instead as a type of energy or light that quickly and easily gets sucked into this vortex, never to be seen again.

There are lots of ways you can imagine weight melting off your body, but I like this imagery a lot. It's almost as if the excess weight is being transformed into life force energy and being stored in your body as a much purer form of energy than fat. You're storing it as invisible, healing life force energy. So imagine the excess weight on your legs, hips, stomach, chest, arms, face, and neck all becoming white light and getting sucked into the energy vortex in your navel, never to be seen again. Feel and imagine yourself sitting there with no excess weight on your body.

STEP 4: CREATE YOUR IDEAL SELF

Now that the fat is melting away and becoming energy, turn your inner attention to your ideal self. Picture your desired body shape, and imagine what it feels like to be sitting inside that perfect shape. Feel your skin tight, muscles toned, belly flat, and a lightness of being. Picture moving through your life in this ideal body: at work, cooking at home, running on the beach, playing a favorite sport, heading out for a date, or eating lunch with friends. As you create these scenes, try to invoke as many senses as possible. If you're imagining yourself at the ocean, hear the waves crashing on the beach, smell and taste the salt water, and feel the sun on your shoulders, the wind in your hair, the sand under your feet, and the cool refreshing water on your ankles. See, imagine, and feel what it's like to have a body that's toned and tight and firm and moving through the scene you've created.

Imagine any work or social events you have planned for the day going smoothly and successfully.

STEP 5: ENVISION COMING DAYS AND MONTHS

After you've imagined scenes from your day-to-day life, turn your attention toward the future. Picture scenarios that you *want* to happen. See yourself becoming fitter, healthier, calmer, more confident, and more desirable. You may want to envision more success in business, more loving relationships, or healthier boundaries. Look ahead days, months, or even years down the road, and see yourself arriving at a place where you've attained your ideal body, shape, and life situation. Maybe you've started a tremendously successful business or you're marrying your ideal partner or you're free from a challenging situation and in a much healthier one. You've healed any chronic issues you may have faced, the excess weight has easily melted off you, and struggle is a thing of the past.

STEP 6: MAGNETIZE YOUR FUTURE

As you see yourself months and years down the road, in your perfect, ideal shape and body, imagine that this future version of you becomes a magnet that's pulling you toward the direction of total success. It's as if your future is pulling you toward it, and you can't resist. You're effortlessly attaining all your dreams and desires. You make the right food choices, the right business choices; you become naturally drawn to movement. Even the most mundane issues of turning left or right on a street, you're now doing because of the magnetic pull of your perfect life. See yourself going through your life from now till that future time, easily getting fitter, healthier, happier, and more successful.

STEP 7: BRING IT BACK TO YOUR BODY AND GET RECHARGED

Finally, bring that bright image of your future self back to your body and imagine that super-successful future self becomes you right now, as you're sitting there. Feel the new you that you've just created charging every cell of your body with success. Whether it's success in weight loss, business, relationships, or whatever your dream, the energy of your beautiful future is charging up your cells and filling you with the energy to achieve your dreams.

And then, just before you open your eyes, feel and affirm that the visualization you've just done will change your life forever. Say to yourself, *With the power of my mind, I've created my ideal body. My excess weight easily and effortlessly melts off me, and I allow myself to achieve success in every area of my life, now and always.*

Once you've finished your visualization, you may want to stay in the extremely pleasurable state of SMART Mode longer and meditate for a while. I know I've really come to enjoy meditation, and I can tell you that the benefits keep coming. So if you feel inclined, simply stay there for a few minutes or longer and continue to breathe into your navel and imagine the ball of light spinning around as you breathe.

However, this isn't necessary. You can simply do the visualization, and all you need is about 10 minutes, from beginning to end. The timeline for a sample visualization might look like this:

Step 1: Get into SMART Mode: 2 to 3 minutes
Step 2: Make Affirmations: 1 to 2 minutes
Step 3: Melt the Weight Off: 1 to 2 minutes
Step 4: Create Your Ideal Self: 1 minute
Step 5: Envision Coming Days and Months: 1 to 2 minutes
Step 6: Magnetize Your Future: 1 minute
Step 7: Bring It Back to Your Body and Get Recharged: 1 minute

Total time: 8–12 minutes

As you practice, you'll become much faster at reaching SMART Mode and then traveling through your visualizations. You'll find yourself sliding into your alpha and theta states much more quickly, and once you've established your affirmations and your future desires, you'll be able visualize at a moment's notice. Once you've done your visualization in SMART mode, it's like a program you've created inside your body. You can then turn that program on during the day simply by thinking about it. It will be like flipping a switch: all the things that you've visualized will come back instantaneously—the fat melting off your body, the success you've imagined, the protection. It's an excellent way of reinforcing your goals and your perfect self.

Again, the purpose of this chapter is to give you all the tools you need to create amazingly effective visualizations on your own. But if this seems a bit much, you can simply listen to the three I've created for you, which you can find at www.TheGabrielMethod .com/visualization-bonus. Or you can record your own visualizations and use them as a guide. Often starting out with guided visualizations is the best way to go. Eventually you'll get to a place where you can easily visualize on your own.

CHAPTER 12

THE GREATER WORLD OF MIND-BODY PRACTICES

The more time you spend visualizing, the more you'll naturally be drawn to other types of mind-body practices, such as meditation, that will contribute to your weight loss success. As I've worked through my weight loss, I've gotten to a point where meditation isn't a chore for me. In fact, it's one of the most pleasurable experiences in my life. I love getting into that calm, relaxed state, and I love feeling my whole body being recharged with energy. Oftentimes I get sudden flashes of inspiration that can be life changing when I'm in a deep meditation.

I've also noticed a direct correlation between the quality of my meditations and the quality of my life. When I have a great meditation session in the morning, I know the rest of my day is going to be enjoyable and productive. I'm calmer, more present, and less reactive, and that equals less stress, more clarity, and more vitality. Meditation unblocks your energy channels and gets your subtle life force flowing. I find that when my energy is flowing, my life is flowing. It's that simple.

Other mind-body practices, such as yoga, tai chi, and qigong, also help reduce stress and contribute to weight loss. They do the same thing for others that meditation does for me, so it's great to keep these practices in mind as you're trying to lose weight.

THE PROOF OF PRACTICE

The practice of yoga has been with us for ages. At the Indus Valley, a site in India that archeologists date to the third millennium B.C., images depict people in various yoga poses. That's quite a testament to yoga's lasting power as a physical and spiritual practice, though it only reached Western shores in the 1890s. It wasn't until a century later that doctors began to recognize its health benefits.

In 1990, Dean Ornish, M.D., founder of the Preventive Medicine Research Institute in Sausalito, California, published in *The Lancet* the results of a lifestyle-change study that included yoga. He found that a whole-person approach combining healing whole foods, yoga, community support, and meditation could actually reverse blockages in the arteries of heart patients. Dr. Ornish's work prompted a flood of studies on the healing power of yoga.[1]

A 2001 study at the University of California, Davis, found that two 90-minute classes a week of hatha-yoga (the most common form taught in the United States) for eight weeks boosted arm and leg strength of the volunteers by as much as 31 percent. And even though they weren't performing the type of exercise we typically think of as aerobically challenging—walking, running, and so on—their muscular endurance increased by 57 percent and their aerobic capacity jumped by almost 10 percent.[2]

Yoga can also help you lose weight. Alan Kristal, Ph.D., associate head of the Cancer Prevention Program in the Public Health Sciences Division at the Hutchinson Center, found that regular yoga practice can help prevent the typical weight gain that occurs in most people in their 40s and 50s. In the study, Kristal and colleagues tracked the health of 15,500 healthy men and women between the ages of 45 and 55. He found that middle-age people who practice yoga gained less weight over a ten-year period than those who did not, and the results were independent of other physical activity and dietary patterns.[3] "We hypothesized that mindfulness—a skill learned either directly or indirectly through yoga—could affect eating behavior," Kristal says.

In another study, he and colleagues interviewed 300 fit people to find out how often they engaged in mindless eating—a risk factor for weight gain. About 40 percent of the people surveyed did yoga regularly. Kristal queried the volunteers about behaviors such as eating when full, noshing in response to environmental cues such as television commercials, or snacking when they felt stressed or upset.[4]

Kristal discovered that the yoga group was much less likely to engage in mindless eating. They also weighed less on average. Adding a yoga practice to any weight loss program could make it more effective, he says. Researchers have also found that other relaxation-based, gentle movement practices, such as tai chi and qigong, produce similar results to those seen from yoga.

Let's look a little more closely at the wealth of research documenting meditation's ability to increase mindfulness, reduce stress, and aid in weight loss. A study from the Duke University Integrative Medicine Center in North Carolina suggests that overweight volunteers lost more weight when they meditated than they did with just diet and exercise alone. The combination of relaxation benefits and improved awareness of physical cues from the body was responsible for the loss, according to the researchers.[5]

The relaxing nature of meditation grants all the benefits of lowering stress, including decreasing cortisol and inflammation, and boosting immune function. But regular meditation will also alter your brain, allowing you to manage future stressful situations with grace and calm. Neurologists at Massachusetts General Hospital and Boston University have found that meditation actually changes the behavior of the amygdala, which you might remember is the seat of aggression and fear in the brain. As the neurologists closely monitored the activity of the amygdala, volunteers looked at images of people who were in positive, negative, or neutral situations. The volunteers then underwent meditation training for two months, after which they viewed another set of negative images.

After regularly practicing meditation, the volunteers reacted much more calmly to the disturbing images. Activity in the amygdala decreased, and the neurologists concluded that meditation improved emotional stability while calming the stress response.[6]

Meditation also helps support your visualization efforts because it can actually improve your ability to visualize. Psychologists at George Mason University in Washington, D.C., showed meditators and nonmeditators a series of detailed images, and then later asked them to identify one of the images among a set of previously unseen images. The meditators were much better at recalling the visual memory task than the nonmeditators were. This, say the researchers, indicates that meditation allows access to greater levels of visuospatial memory resources.[7] Recalling visual memories is extremely useful when practicing visualization. You may want to recall a pleasurable scene when you were fit, happy, and healthy. The better able you are to imagine these kinds of positive memories, the more effective your visualizations will be.

THE EASTERN EXPLANATION

Neurologists are finding that mind-body practices produce many physiological benefits, including altering the expression of genes in our DNA as well as a whole host of cellular and hormonal changes. Eastern and traditional medical professionals attribute the benefits of mind-body practices to another source: chi or qi, a subtle energy current of life force that runs through the body. In Ayurvedic medicine, it's referred to as prana.

Many medical professionals scoff at the idea of chi, but we didn't even know we had radio waves until a few hundred years ago. In fact, there are lots of invisible forms of energy that we're discovering all the time. As we develop instruments to detect the subtle waves, they are "discovered."

In the visual spectrum, our eyes can only see certain frequencies corresponding to the color spectrum from red to violet. But we also know there is a whole range of other energies in that very same spectrum that we can't see, such as radio waves, microwaves, gamma ray, X-rays, and so on. All these subtle energies have always existed, but we didn't know they were there until recently because we couldn't "see" them and we didn't have instruments to detect them.

In the same way, we have a subtle life force energy current that runs through our bodies that we can't detect with our senses, but it is there nonetheless. Eastern medicine has been studying this subtle life force energy for thousands of years, and, according to experts in the field, our chi is at the essence of the mind-body connection.

Ever wonder how thought creates movement? To me, this is one of the greatest miracles in the world and something that has always puzzled me. How does a thought—an invisible, nonphysical notion—translate to movement in our bodies? We think, *I want to pick up that apple,* and that invisible thought somehow creates movement. Neurons fire and nerves stimulate muscle contractions in an amazingly complex and coordinated sequence and the apple gets picked up. Truly miraculous!

Chinese medicine has an explanation. Our thoughts are a force. Not a strong enough force to move matter—at least not for most of us—but a force strong enough to move chi energy. The chi energy then creates an energetic ripple that affects the electrons in our brain cells. That causes our brain cells to "fire," sending messages to other brain cells, which results in nerves firing and muscles contracting. So our life force energy, a subtle form of energy that responds to our desires, is the interface between thought and movement.

This subtle life force energy circulates through the body along discrete, invisible pathways, just like blood travels through arteries and veins. Known in acupuncture as meridians, or nadis, these pathways keep the body working smoothly. In traditional forms of medicine, disease originates when blockages occur in these energy channels. Treating disease requires removing the energy blockage and restoring the flow. That's what acupuncturists are doing with needles: they're unblocking your energy channels.

You're at your healthiest and most vibrant when your energy channels are open and flowing freely. When you have blockages, your entire body will suffer as a result. You'll feel exhausted, you'll be stressed, and you'll get sick. All of this can lead to the activation of your FAT programs, so getting your life force pathways open and flowing is the best way to create health, stay fit, and boost your vitality.

Our energy channels become blocked through fear, negativity, and stress. The pathways constrict, trapping healthy energy and allowing negative emotions and energies to dominate. Treating these troubles is possible using any of the mind-body practices we've discussed. They all improve the flow of this life force energy.

Dawson Church, Ph.D., the energy researcher and author of *The Genie in Your Genes,* says, "The body's connective tissue system is a giant liquid crystal semiconductor," which means that when you stretch it through yoga or activate it through the gentle movements of tai chi or qigong, you're improving your life force energy flow. He also goes on to say:

> Studies show that points on the life force meridians have much lower electrical resistance (averaging 10,000 ohms at the center of the point) when compared to the surrounding skin (which averages a much higher 3,000,000 ohms). Among other characteristics, acupuncture points propagate acoustic sound better than does the surrounding skin. They also emit small amounts of light and greater amounts of carbon dioxide. When the points are stimulated with a low-frequency current, the body responds by producing endorphins and cortisol. When they are stimulated with a higher-frequency current, the body produces serotonin and norepinephrine. When the surrounding skin receives the same current, these neurochemicals are not produced.[8]

So it's clear that cutting-edge medical science is recognizing the validity of the 5,000-year-old study of chi energy, acupuncture meridians, and our subtle life force energy channels.

What's common to nearly all mind-body practices is that they use visualization and/or breathing techniques to direct life force energy to different parts of the body and unblock energy channels. Remember that life force energy is moved and controlled by your mind. In yoga, tai chi, and qigong, you're using breathing, visualization, and gentle movement or stretching to direct life force through the body. In guided meditations, you're using breathing and/or visualization to circulate your life force energy. As you direct life force energy to various parts of your body, it clears out blockages, so that your channels are open and flowing.

On a very practical note, when your energy channels are open, and your chi is flowing, you simply have more energy, which means you will have fewer junk food cravings. One of the reasons we crave empty-calorie junk food is because we're chronically exhausted, and one of the reasons we're exhausted is our life force energy isn't flowing. When you get your energy channels flowing, you have an entirely different way to energize your body, so you are not as dependent on food.

VISUALIZATION TO UNBLOCK ENERGY CHANNELS

To help unblock your energy channels and circulate healing life force vitality throughout your body, you can use visualization in addition to the mind-body practices we've discussed above. In this visualization, you're using the power of your mind to direct life force energy throughout your body, nourishing and healing your entire body.

> Sit straight with your chin slightly down, so that your spine is like one long line from the bottom of your spine to the base of your head. Keep your mouth closed if possible and comfortable and let your tongue slightly touch the roof of your mouth. Have your hands gently folded together on your lap.
>
> Now take a deep breath in, and then let that breath out and relax. Just imagine there's a ball of light in your navel and it's circulating around. And it's getting brighter and brighter, and as it's circulating around it's pulling energy up from the earth. Energy is coming from the earth, into your feet, and into your shins and ankles, and into your calves, and into your knees, and

it's circulating around your legs and your bones, and it's going into your thighs, and it's going into your pelvis, and it's going into that ball of energy in your navel.

And as this ball is pulling energy up from the earth and spinning around your navel, imagine that it's also pulling energy down from the sky. That energy is filling your head with bright white light, and if you touch your tongue to the roof of your mouth, you might feel the trickle as that energy goes into your tongue and into your throat, filling your throat with bright white light. And you feel it move into your heart, filling your heart and your lungs with bright white light. And then down into your navel.

So your whole body is being filled with light. Energy from the earth is coming into your legs. Energy from the sky is coming into your head, and it is all meeting in your navel. And your navel is spinning around with bright white light, getting brighter and brighter and brighter. And this ball of white light is getting bigger and bigger so that it's filling your whole stomach and your pelvis and your thighs and your chest and your shoulders and your shins and your ankles and your head. It's getting bigger and bigger and brighter and brighter. And it's above your head and it's below your feet and you're covered in a big ball of bright white light. And every cell of your body is being bathed in this bright white light.

Imagine the energy starting to move from one arm, into your hand and then into the other hand and up the other arm. So in this way, energy is flowing around your arms, as well. So now you have a ball of light in your navel that's circulating like a galaxy of light or a vortex. It's pulling energy up from the earth, into your legs and into the vortex. It's pulling energy down from the sky, into your head and chest and into the energy vortex. Energy is also circulating around your arms, and your entire body is covered by an ever-growing ball of beautiful bright white light.

Now just sit for a few minutes, with your back straight, your tongue lightly touching the roof of your mouth, and your hands folded together on your lap. Breathe into and out of your navel and imagine that while you breathe in, the spiral turns faster, like a pinwheel in the wind, and as you breathe out, the spiral turns faster, as well. Don't worry about which direction it turns, either way is fine, you are circulating energy through your body. Just spend a few minutes breathing into and out of your navel and imagining the energy circulating and moving in all directions as you breathe. See the energy coming up from the earth, down from the sky, all converging in your navel and growing into an ever-brighter, ever-larger ball of energy.

When you're ready to finish, imagine the vortex of light in your navel sucking up all the excess light that is coming up from the earth, down from the sky, and circulating all around your body. Imagine it all gets sucked into this circulating vortex and stored there as life force vitality that you can use anytime you want or need.

Doing mind-body practices, including visualization, not only helps you open your energy channels and improve your life force; they can also help you increase your intuition, which, as we'll talk about in the next chapter, can also be extremely useful for weight loss.

CHAPTER 13

INTUITIVE WEIGHT LOSS

On one of my favorite bike rides, there is a short but steep hill on a dirt road in farm country just past some local wineries. Although the hill only takes about two or three minutes to climb, it's so intense that I feel a tremendous sense of accomplishment when I reach the top.

I usually celebrate by raising my hands in the air and letting myself fly down the other side of the hill without my hands on the handlebars. Maybe that's not the best idea, but it's fun. I feel so alive when I'm sailing down that hill.

One day, after reaching the top, I was about to do my celebratory coast down the other side, when a little voice inside my head said, *No. Don't do that. Keep your hands on the bars.* I listened, and right after this intuition struck me, a six-foot-tall kangaroo came out of the woods and charged right at me. He wasn't trying to attack me. Kangaroos are like 200-pound squirrels: when they're startled, they'll just charge across the road. While hitting a squirrel can make you feel bad, smashing into a kangaroo is a whole other story. He was just trying to get to the other side of the road, and he wasn't too bothered by the fact that he might have to trample me in the process.

I was already moving at full speed when he charged. I had less than a millisecond to respond. I swerved quickly and started heading for the far side of the road. Thankfully there were no cars. I also slammed on my brakes and felt the back of my bike lifting as I went into a skid. I managed to turn the bike almost completely around and land in a ditch with nothing but some scrapes from sliding on the road.

I hesitate to imagine what would have happened if I had my hands in the air, like I usually do. There's no way I could have controlled my bike, and I would have crashed headfirst into that kangaroo. While kangaroos are normally peaceful animals, they do have sharp talons on their hind legs and routinely disembowel dogs or other predators when threatened.

So what was that little voice inside my head that saved my life? And what made me listen to it?

THE VOICE WITHIN

Maybe you've had a lifesaving experience like mine. We've all heard of remarkable stories where "chance" saves people's lives and changes them forever. This is our intuition, and, although it's not been widely studied, it's an amazing asset that we are all born with and something we can develop and cultivate.

If you're not sure whether intuition is for real, consider this quote: "Research in human pattern recognition and decision-making suggests that there is a 'sixth sense' through which humans can detect and act on unique patterns without consciously and intentionally analyzing them." Where's the quote from? The Office of Naval Research for the United States Department of Defense.[1] That's correct; the U.S. Navy's research department is so interested in developing this sixth sense that it has begun a $3.85 million four-year research project into the understanding of intuition.

The reason the Navy is interested in intuition is because of the overwhelming number of soldiers and sailors who've made lifesaving decisions based on a hunch. In one case, a staff sergeant saved the lives of 17 civilians in a café because he sensed something odd about a would-be bomber. An entire Canadian company of soldiers survived an ambush in Afghanistan based on their intuition that they were wandering into a possible trap. Belief in intuition permeates the business world, as well. A poll from PR

Week and Burson-Marsteller suggests that most CEOs rely on their intuition when making important decisions.[2]

But polls and anecdotal stories aren't the only reason the U.S. Navy wants to learn more about the sixth sense. The stress research institute HeartMath in California has looked carefully into the phenomenon of intuition. In one study, they had subjects sit in front of a blank computer screen. Occasionally, the computer would flash an image. Some were pleasant scenes, of nature, for example, while others were upsetting, such as a photo of an autopsy. As the images flashed by, the HeartMath researchers carefully monitored the volunteers' brains and hearts to see when and how they might respond to the images.

An initial surprising finding was that the heart responded before the brain did: the first reaction came not from the mind as you might expect, but from the heart. But far more remarkable was the fact that both the heart and the brain responded *before* the disturbing image even appeared. The computer was set to produce the images in random order, yet the volunteers *knew* whether the image would be pleasant or upsetting milliseconds before it appeared on the screen. Based on the results, the researchers concluded that "the body's perceptual apparatus is continuously scanning the future."[3]

Your intuition is very real indeed, as you've probably suspected from incidents in your own life. It's something we are all born with but we lose over time. It atrophies, like a muscle that's never used. Our society simply doesn't encourage the development and use of intuition, so it just gets weaker.

What's different about this sixth sense from the other five senses is that it's a nonphysical sense, and therefore not bound by time and space. With our five senses, we can only perceive what's directly around us or touching us; we can only see, hear, smell, taste, and touch what's physically happening in the moment. Our sixth sense lets us perceive things that will happen, have happened, or are happening somewhere else in the world.

Remember that quantum physics teaches us that all time exists now. That means that the past, present, and future are all happening now. We just can't perceive the past and future with our five senses, the same way we can't perceive chi energy with our five senses. But mathematically, we know it's true that all time exists in the eternal present.

Our intuition is not bound by time and space, so it can accurately assess the future, simply because the future is, in actuality, happening as we speak. That's why subjects in the HeartMath study were able to sense an upsetting image that was going to appear on the screen *before it actually happened.*

INTUITION, SAFETY, AND WEIGHT LOSS

As you might imagine, having a developed sixth sense is one of the best ways to help you feel safe in your day-to-day life. Imagine having a developed, reliable intuition that always knew what was going to happen to you in the next few moments, days, or years? You could be walking home from work and your intuition might tell you to turn left instead of right. You might think, *That's ridiculous. I always walk home turning right here; it's a shorter and more direct route.* But what you may not know—what you have no way of knowing—is that if you turn right a piano will land on your head. Your intuition can pick this up, but if you're not able to hear the message or you don't listen, you can't benefit from the information.

Melinda, a Gabriel Method coach and intuitive healer, experienced firsthand just how powerful listening to your intuition can be. She was in a movie theater in Aurora, Colorado, in 2012 about to watch a midnight screening of *The Dark Knight Rises* when all of a sudden she felt an extreme uneasiness in her stomach. She knew something wasn't right. She could feel it intuitively, and she left the theater at once. That was on the ill-fated night of the Aurora, Colorado, shootings. After she left, a gunman launched tear gas into the theater and then proceeded to gun down innocent victims: 12 people were killed and 70 wounded. Her highly developed intuition kept her out of harm's way.

We place so much emphasis on knowledge and intelligence, but they both pale in comparison to intuition when it comes to safety. If you have a fully developed intuition, you can relax and let your intuition guide you. It will tell you who to do business with, what stocks to buy, where to buy real estate, who you can trust, and how to stay out of danger. You'll be directed to your soul mates, teachers, business partners, and true friends. The list of benefits is endless, and it's all courtesy of your own intuitive guidance. From a weight loss perspective, you'll be guided to the foods that heal your digestive system and reduce inflammation, the right support community, the right fitness coach, the right guides for inspiration, and anything else you might need to help you along the way. All this is possible by merely tapping into a sense perception mechanism that most of us don't even realize we have.

So how do you strengthen your intuition? Wouldn't it be nice if you could develop a way to be more aware of the world around you—not just to keep you safe from threats, but for the opportunities as well? There's a straightforward way to strengthen your intuition.

MUSCLE BUILDING FOR INTUITION

When a child is born with a lazy eye, the ophthalmologist will recommend an eye patch for the good eye. Why is that? The muscles in the lazy eye are weak, and as the child relies more on the good eye, its muscles get stronger and stronger and the lazy eye gets weaker and weaker. The patch forces the child to focus and control the lazy eye, developing the muscles of that eye, so it can compete with the stronger one. Eventually, both eyes will be able to work in tandem.

Our atrophied sixth sense is much like a lazy third eye. It's gotten so weak that it can't compete with the stronger five senses that we've come to rely on. So the way to strengthen your sixth sense is to put a "patch" on your other five senses. That's exactly what's happening when you're meditating. Meditation is the act of being awake and aware and *not* using your five senses. As you sit quietly with your eyes closed, you begin to perceive the world and your surroundings through a different sense perception. You begin strengthening your sixth sense.

Numerous studies demonstrate that the brains of meditators gain mass in areas related to emotional sensitivity. My experiences have led me to believe that meditation is like a muscle-building exercise for your intuition, allowing you to make better decisions throughout your day and your life.

Eventually, after days and months of daily practice, your sixth sense gets strong enough to work in concert with your other five senses, so that during the day, as you go about your business, you're perceiving the world with all six senses.

VISUALIZATION TO DEVELOP INTUITION

Here's a quick visualization you can do to help develop your intuition and strengthen your lazy "third" eye.

In SMART Mode (see pages 20–21), imagine breathing in and out of your forehead. Just imagine that as you are inhaling, you are actually inhaling from your forehead and as you are exhaling you are exhaling from that same point. Imagine you are in an ocean of white light and you are breathing that white light in and out of your forehead. As you breathe the light into your forehead, it fills your head and then your entire body with white light. Continue doing this for a few minutes, just inhaling and exhaling white light into your body from your forehead. You may start to notice some light or patterns developing in your forehead. If you do, just allow them to be there and don't pay too much attention to them.

As you continue to breathe through your forehead, imagine that you have a large eye in the middle of your forehead that opens up and starts seeing. Imagine that this eye can clearly see your future and imagine your most perfect future, in the coming months and years. See yourself in your perfect, ideal shape, getting fitter and fitter as days go by. See your career and your relationships improving. See it all as one long timeline stretching into the future. Now feel that this eye that has opened up in your forehead is guiding you to your most perfect ideal body and ideal life. Feel and affirm that throughout your day, every day, every step you make will be guided by this intuition toward creating the vision of your perfect life that you've just created.

Then just remain in that state of breathing white light into and out of your body from your forehead for as long as you like.

The reason why most of us are so frantic much of the time is because no matter how smart we are, we don't know what's going to happen. That makes intuition one of the greatest gifts we have.

Your intuition may lead you to dramatic life changes. You may drop your current job and go back to school. You may move to California and start growing sprouts. Your decisions may not seem logical at first, but you'll find that living by your intuition means you'll meet the right people, you'll be in the right place at the right time, and you'll be living the life you're "meant" to live. You'll start to relax and trust your guidance. If you look at successful people, there's always some chance meeting or opportunity that they were able to take advantage of that is only apparent in hindsight. These changes may not make sense in the moment, but when you look back, you'll be able to connect the dots to see why it happened.

Once you realize how amazing an asset intuition is and that you have the ability to strengthen your intuition at will, you'll want to spend increasingly more time developing it. Your intuition will help you feel safer and that will lower your stress levels and allow you to lose weight much more easily, as well as guide you to your most ideal life.

Next up, let's talk about another issue that really aids in weight loss: nutrition. This discussion comes not with the idea of counting calories, but with a focus on how to best use food to energize, nourish, love, and support your body while you're going through this transformation. This will not only fill you with the nutrients your body needs but also provide the ideal hormonal environment that will support sustainable weight loss.

CHAPTER 14

NUTRITION DEMYSTIFIED

You may be wondering why it's only now that we're getting around to talking about food. This might seem a little late in the process, but as I'm sure you're already aware, food is just one small part of the weight loss equation. We all know people who eat as much as they like of whatever they want and never gain a pound. And we also all know people who are constantly dieting and starving themselves and yet can't seem to lose any weight. People who fall into the latter category know what it's like to deny cravings day and night, living every day as a battle between willpower and insatiable hunger.

As we've discussed throughout the book, when it comes to weight loss, the real issue is hormones and hormonal balance, and this extends well beyond food. Your thoughts, your beliefs, your sleep, and even the air you breathe contribute to your chemistry and hormones. Food is one of many mind-body factors that can influence your hormonal balance and your weight.

As you may have already found if you've started the process, reducing stress and resolving emotional traumas through visualization creates a chemical shift in your body that facilitates weight loss. There are still many ways you can alter your diet that will help you lose weight sustainably; however, the focus has to be on hormonal balance, not simply calories. You'll also do wonders for your health, your mood, and your life by following a few simple guidelines when you eat—and also by ignoring the supposed hard-and-fast rule of dieting.

FORGET "CALORIES IN, CALORIES OUT"

While the words *just eat less* are usually the first thing out of a nutritional expert's mouth, they're just plain wrong. It might seem logical to assume that eating less and exercising more is the only way to lose weight, but it's a faulty premise. The theory is what Dr. Ron Rosedale, founder of the Carolina Center of Metabolic Medicine, calls "kindergarten medicine." Many biochemical researchers are only now beginning to understand the enormous complexity of the body's metabolic processes and that the idea of eating fewer calories is not the only way to lose weight. Hormonal balance is the new model, and the very first doctor to devise a strategy that was based on this model was the late Dr. Atkins.

Although I complain about Dr. Atkins's treatment of me, he was truly revolutionary in his approach to weight loss in one sense: he successfully disproved the age-old adage that weight loss is simply a matter of "calories in, calories out."

As early as the 1960s, Dr. Robert Atkins suspected there were problems with this equation. Atkins understood how carbohydrates raised insulin levels and how that could lead to the body generating more fat stores. Remember, insulin is the fat-making hormone, so when insulin levels are elevated, your body generates more fat. Also, when insulin levels are elevated, the body loses the ability to burn fat because insulin prevents the body from secreting fat-burning hormones. So we end up in a state where we are perpetually making fat and never burning it.

Dr. Atkins reasoned that if we don't eat carbohydrates, insulin levels won't rise and we'll generate and store less fat; we might even burn fat more easily. When he tried feeding volunteers a fat-and-protein-based diet, Atkins found that, sure enough, people could eat as much as they wanted, avoid counting calories, yet still avoid gaining weight. In fact, they could shed pounds eating mostly red meat, bacon, and butter—at least for a while.

Using the high-fat and high-protein diet, Atkins was able to conclusively show that calories in, calories out was a fallacy, even though it took almost 30 years before mainstream scientists accepted his findings. However, the Atkins Diet is still one-dimensional. Even though eating this way can keep insulin levels down, the diet promotes inflammation and digestive troubles that eventually lead to insulin resistance and a rise in insulin levels. The inflammation also causes leptin resistance, triggering insatiable hunger. Ultimately, people who lose weight with Atkins often gain it back as they do with any one-dimensional program.

Other hormone-based diets try to address the issue of elevated insulin levels and insulin and leptin resistance. But they're all limited in scope because they fail to look at the myriad influences behind these hormonal problems. One example comes from Dr. Robert H. Lustig, University of California–San Francisco professor of pediatrics in the division of endocrinology. Lustig is a strong advocate of a low-fructose diet, and he has demonstrated with detailed biochemical equations how fructose, a sugar derived from fruit, causes insulin resistance in the liver and elevates free fatty acids in the bloodstream. This professor is very convincing when he states that he'd rather eat a piece of bread than a piece of fruit because bread has less fructose.

But the metabolism of fructose is extremely complicated and not yet fully understood. All the studies that demonstrate the adverse effects of fructose have been with done with a highly processed and concentrated form of fructose called high fructose corn syrup (HFCS). Not all fructose is digested the same. Sometimes fructose is digested in the large intestine and sometimes in the liver, and, to date, no one knows why this is so. There's still lots we don't know about the sugar. While it's crystal clear that HFCS leads to insulin resistance, leptin resistance, and weight gain, it's not clear at all whether the same is true for the fructose in fruit. I've never seen a study in laboratory animals or humans that proves that fruit will make you fat. I'm going to go out on a limb and say you can feed a rat all the fruit it can eat and there's a good chance it won't gain any weight or suffer the metabolic consequences that it would if it were eating large quantities of HFCS.

Once again it comes down to the issue of processed versus real. Bread causes an exaggerated insulin response in the bloodstream, much greater than that of fruit, and it leads to leptin and insulin resistance—the very problems caused by HFCS. Even worse, bread contains gluten that irritates the bowels, causes inflammation, and leads to the release of inflammatory hormones that also cause leptin and insulin resistance. The conclusion that bread is better than fruit simply because bread has less fructose is an untested one and one that I wholeheartedly disagree with. Fruit also has live enzymes that assist in digestion, lots of antioxidants, and nutrients that are essential to the body and to weight loss.

While you might think the answer is avoiding all types of sugar, in my experience, stress and toxins are usually the triggers for the metabolic syndromes that cause leptin and insulin resistance. When you address these factors, the body becomes much more tolerant of sugars.

SOME SIMPLE GUIDELINES

After you address the stress and fear that are turning on your FAT programs, you start to understand that the premise behind these diets that focus on what to eat and what not to eat becomes unstable.

In fact the whole question of whether to eat fats, carbohydrates, or proteins is a nonissue. What we need to focus on is the *type* of fats, carbohydrates, and proteins. The right type of fat is one of the best things you can put in your body and will help reverse the chemical syndromes that cause weight gain, allowing you to lose weight much more easily. The wrong type of fat will do the exact opposite. The same is true for carbohydrates and proteins. Your goal is to consume fats, proteins, and carbohydrates that reduce stress, toxins, inflammation, and leptin and insulin resistance.

You might think this sounds complicated, but actually it's quite simple. A good rule of thumb is, if nature made it, it's good for you; if it's man-made, it's bad. Sure, there are exceptions to this rule, but generally speaking, if you want to identify the foods that are best for you and your weight loss goals, don't worry about calories, carbs, fats, or proteins. The simplest criteria is whether the food is processed or not.

Live, organic nuts, seeds, salads, vegetables, most fruits, cold-pressed nut and seed oils, herbs, spices, and unprocessed animal proteins all nourish your body without causing excessive insulin levels, digestive stress, or inflammation. They contain more nutrients than processed foods do, more digestive enzymes, and more essential friendly bacteria. Your digestive system can easily extract nutrients from these foods. As a result, you feel more nourished, have more energy, and won't feel as hungry. Your cells will function better and become more sensitive to fat-regulating hormones, and you'll lose weight much easier.

Processed foods are often stripped of valuable nutrients, and they can contain artificial sweeteners, colorings, and flavor enhancers, refined vegetable oils, and genetically modified ingredients. They may also contain pesticides, fungicides, and herbicides that disrupt the hormonal balance in your body, leading to digestive troubles, inflammation, and exaggerated insulin levels that trigger your FAT programs. Because they're nutritionally deficient, you'll feel hungry even after you've had plenty to eat. These foods are also highly addictive. Many processed foods also cause wild blood sugar fluctuations that eventually cause your body to lose the ability to regulate blood sugar and burn fat.

In the highly competitive trillion-dollar food industry, the motivation for processing foods isn't to nourish your body or make you healthier. The motivation is to create foods that are cheaper to manufacture, cheaper to ship, last longer on the shelf, and make you want to eat more of them. And unfortunately, none of those incentives have your body's best interest at heart.

To help guide you to the best foods, ask yourself this question: "Could I find this food I'm eating right now, in this form, thousands of years ago?" If the answer is yes, you're nourishing yourself and allowing your body to become more efficient at losing weight. If the answer is no, you're not nourishing your body, you're nourishing a multinational food conglomerate instead. It really is that simple.

Now, you may not be craving real foods initially. But that changes over time. There are several reasons why we crave junk food, including leptin and insulin resistance, addictions, blood sugar problems, and parasites. So simply start by adding real foods as much as possible. In addition, I recommend adding fermented/cultured foods to heal digestion and foods high in omega-3 fatty acids to help reduce inflammation and help reverse leptin and insulin resistance. If you're looking for delicious recipes that incorporate real foods, please visit www.TheGabriel Method.com/cookbook-preview1.

The real solution to losing weight is already in your hands. Take the time to visualize daily, and you'll soon solve your weight issues. But you can support your body's desires to be thin by making better choices when you eat, and these simple recipes can show you how.

MAKING THE CHANGE

If you've been eating a lot of convenience foods, processed foods, and fast foods, making many of these changes to your diet will be rough going at first. Please remember that you shouldn't try to toss out your diet overnight—you won't last too long if you're practicing nothing but denial. Plus, it's likely that you're addicted to the extreme seasoning you get in processed foods. They're usually loaded with toxic fats and sugars and artificial flavor enhancers to help stimulate your appetite and encourage addiction.

When you first start eating more live raw foods and quality animal proteins, just add them to your diet. Go ahead and have a cheeseburger if that's what you're craving, but first prepare and eat a big salad sprinkled with chia seeds and a chia or flaxseed oil salad dressing, because they're high in omega-3s. Also it would be great if the meat were organic and derived from grass-fed cattle, as there will be fewer pesticides, hormones, and preservatives and the fat will be much healthier. Maybe put the cheeseburger on top of the salad. That's what I do and I find that to be enormously satisfying. The thought of eating the bun is very much repulsive to me at this point, but there was a time when I couldn't imagine feeling satisfied eating a burger without the bun. Once the addiction is broken, the bun holds no more allure than a piece of Styrofoam.

As the stress in your life reduces, your digestive health increases, and your body is better nourished, you'll find that you start to crave the live "real" foods more, and dead, toxic, highly processed "fake" foods will lose their appeal entirely.

You can also use visualization to help develop the habit of eating, loving, and craving healthy and nutritious foods. Anything you imagine yourself doing, you will be much more likely to do in real life.

Once you're in SMART Mode (see pages 20–21), picture yourself becoming hungry during your day, whether you're at work or at home. Imagine that you're craving and eating real, live, healthy, vibrant, nutritious foods. See a plate in front of you. See how beautiful the food looks. Imagine it vibrating with life force vitality. See lots of different types of real foods, such as green leafy salads, yellow peppers, purple onions, red cherry tomatoes, succulent mangoes, papayas, berries, and healthy crunchy nuts and seeds full of essential fatty acids and quality proteins. All these foods are beautifully displayed on your plate. Imagine the wonderful smell of the food. Now picture tasting the food as it bursts with flavor and vitality. Taste the crunch and crackle and soft, sweet, savory flavors as they tingle your taste buds with delight.

Feel the food going into your body and nourishing every single cell in your body. Imagine that your body feels calm, centered, energized, and deeply satisfied. Then imagine having energy and vitality throughout the day as a result of the amazing foods you are eating. Hear every cell of your body saying at the same time the words, "This food is nourishing my body. I love beautiful, live, healthy, vibrant, natural foods. I am nourished and satisfied." Then imagine any excess weight just melting off your body thanks to the vital nourishment that you are providing.

CHAPTER 15

CREATING THE LIFE OF YOUR DREAMS

We've learned a lot about visualization in this book and how it can help you lose weight, but I'd like to take it one step further right now and talk about how you can use visualization to also help you create your ideal life. The two are very much interrelated, because sometimes your life is the problem. For example, the wrong job or a dysfunctional relationship can cause stress that will cause weight gain. So by using visualization to help you achieve your ideal life, you are also helping to solve your weight problems as well.

A lot of inspirational speakers talk about "The Law of Attraction," which is basically using visualization and the power of your thinking to manifest your ideal life. That is, that our minds are like a magnetic force that helps attract to us the experiences we focus on. Jack Canfield describes how he imagined selling 100,000 copies of his book *Chicken Soup for the Soul* in the first year and how that actually came to pass. Jim Carrey, as we talked about, wrote himself a check for 10 million dollars for "acting services rendered," dated it three years into the future and then was actually paid that amount. There are hundreds of amazing stories like this of super successful people using visualization in this way to create their lives.

Many people who are inspired by these stories try visualization for manifesting their ideal life and are frustrated with the results, because they are not exactly as they had envisioned. While there could be any number of reasons for this, I think one of the reasons why they are not getting their desired results might be because their visualization skills are not yet fully developed.

In the same way that we have to learn how to communicate with our bodies using appropriate visual imagery, we have to learn how to communicate our desires to life as well. Just like with your body, it's the images that you have in your head that will influence the outcomes you receive. For example, you may hate your boss and want another job. If you have a dialogue going on in your head that's something like "I hate my boss. He's such a jerk. He's ripping me off," what you're picturing all day is your boss and that's the image you're using the power of your mind to attract. You're also picturing him with intense negative emotion. So if there is such a thing as an attractive law in the universe and you're spending the vast majority of your day picturing this one person in your life and you're doing so with intense negative emotions, it will be much more likely that life will give you more of your boss and the negative feelings associated with him, which is the exact opposite to the result that you want.

That doesn't mean the law of attraction doesn't work; it just means that you haven't yet learned how to effectively communicate your desire. What you need to do is focus on what it is you *do* want: a better job in a better working environment. Imagine this during your visualizations, when your mind is calm, clear, and focused. Then during the day, continue to have the image of the positive outcome that you've just created in your head, instead of the dialogue of hate and resentment surrounding your current situation. By doing this, you'll send a much more clear and consistent message to the universe.

As you learn how to talk to your body in symbols, you'll get better at learning how to talk to the attractive forces of the universe in symbols, too, which is great. As I mentioned before, visualization is like a muscle that gets stronger with use. One of the added benefits of practicing visualization every day for weight loss is that you'll be strengthening your "manifesting muscle" on a daily basis, to the point where you can also achieve more consistent results in manifesting your ideal life.

Law of Attraction enthusiasts claim that our minds are a creative force that attracts to us whatever it is we think about or imagine. If that's true, even to a small degree, doesn't it make sense that the more powerful your mind is and the better you are at visualizing your desired results, the better you'll be at applying this law?

I'm still undecided about the extent to which the law of attraction affects our life. There's no doubt in my mind that there's something to it, but I know I spent a lot of time and energy thinking about Suzanne Somers as a kid and so far nothing's come of that ;-) But in all seriousness I have had some amazing successes using visualization to create my life; so much so that at this point I'm really careful about what I visualize happening.

I remember when I first lost weight I was at the Crown Theatre in Burswood, Perth, attending a talk of a well-known speaker. The place was packed with more than 1,000 people in attendance. The thought occurred to me that one day I would like to be up on this very stage presenting to a sold-out audience. The next day I imagined myself on that stage presenting to a full house. I imagined an explosion of light coming out of me toward the audience while I delivered a powerful speech that the audience loved and got tremendous benefit from.

I included this image in my visualization on a daily basis. I would only hold the image in my head for about 30 seconds, but I did so at the end of my meditation when I was in a very deep state of focus. A few months later I received a call from someone who invited me to speak in Perth at a "weight loss super conference." At that point, I hadn't been on stage or spoken about the Gabriel Method, except to small gatherings in people's houses. It was the first speaking engagement I had ever been invited to.

I asked him where the talk was being held and he said the Burswood Theatre. Sure enough I was up on stage exactly as I had imagined, delivering my message to a highly enthusiastic audience. The energy that was coming out of me was something I had never experienced before. It was nothing short of explosive. After the talk, there was a line of hundreds of people waiting to speak with me and to have me sign their books. So many people wanted to meet me that they had to postpone the next talk by two hours.

The same thing happened with the publishing of this book. I had wanted to work with Hay House, because they're the leader in mind-body wellness and I felt intuitively that they were the right publisher for this message. My team and I had no luck reaching them through the channels we'd used on other books, which is understandable as they are very much in demand. So I turned to visualization and imagined Hay House publishing my next book and having it completely change the way the world approaches health and weight loss.

Once again I included it into my daily practice for about 30 seconds a day, and within a few weeks I got a call from my business partner saying we had just won a contest, and the prize was lunch with the president of Hay House. I met with him and the rest is history.

These are just a few examples from my life, but the daily cause-and-effect relationship between what I imagine happening and what actually happens in my life can be pretty miraculous sometimes. So is there something special about me that allows me to access this mysterious creative power? Not at all. I just happen to have worked out that visualization muscle.

There's nothing special or mysterious about that; it's simply the result of daily practice. A power lifter doesn't develop huge muscles overnight; it takes time. The reason he can lift several hundred pounds more than most people is because he's spent a lot of time developing his muscles. In the same way, years of daily visualization practice have made my powers of focus and concentration much stronger.

And that's exactly what will happen with you, when you start strengthening your own visualization/manifestation muscles. As you get stronger from daily practice, you'll notice an amazing cause-and-effect relationship between your visualizations and the people/events/things that appear in your life. If you want more loving relationships, more abundance, success in business, to win a competition, or to achieve a certain goal, simply imagine yourself, while in SMART Mode, being in the desired situation or accomplishing the goal.

If the results are not immediate, keep in mind that it might take a while for you to get to the place where your manifesting potential is strong enough. But you might have amazing results, too. You never know and you certainly have nothing to lose by trying. For those of us who have tapped into this creative principle, visualization becomes a way of life. It's just understood that part of creating what you want in life is to visualize. Sure, we might work hard to achieve our goals, but it all starts with a vision.

16 WEEKS TO TOTAL TRANSFORMATION

If you're really motivated—or would like additional guidance—you can follow my 16 Weeks to Total Transformation Program. The idea is that for 16 weeks, you'll incorporate visualization into your life regularly in an effort to combat stress and change bad habits. You'll also work to change what you eat so you are as supported as possible in your efforts for weight loss.

Virtually every beneficial aspect of visualization that we've talked about in this book is incorporated into this 16-week transformational experience. Don't worry if you're doing everything right or if the program is working. The more you visualize, the more it will work. Eventually you'll get to a place where you'll know for sure that it's working because you'll find that you're simply less hungry, crave healthier foods, have more energy, and your clothes are getting looser.

You'll also find after a while that your mind will become very calm while you're listening, and your body will feel energized and relaxed. At that point you'll start to feel tremendous after your visualizations. Then you're hooked! It will no longer be an effort or a chore to practice visualization. You'll look forward to it as soon as you get up and you may even want to stay in that calm, relaxed, pleasurable, meditative state for a while after the visualization is over. I sometimes sit and visualize and then meditate for long periods of time in the morning. Not because I think I should, but simply because it feels so amazing and I know that I'm reaping so many positive benefits. But I started, exactly as I'm asking you to start, by simply listening to a seven- to ten-minute visualization first thing in the morning, every morning. So let's just get into the program.

Do Your Visualizations

Every night—or as often as you can—listen to the evening visualization. And every morning try the visualizations below. I've set up a week-by-week plan for you to follow, but feel free to mix and match the weekly visualizations as needed. If you want to address emotional trauma right off the bat, for example, start there. Or maybe you really want to target specific food addictions. While it doesn't matter which order (or even which visualization) you listen in, it is important to have the week's worth of repetition. This will help reinforce the new neural pathways. And remember, there's no wrong way to do these. As long as you're visualizing your perfect life and body daily, on a daily basis, you'll be reaping the benefits.

Week 1: Believe Your Body Wants to Be Thin (pages 156–159)

Week 2: Nourish Your Body (pages 159–161)

Week 3: Reduce Stress (page 162–165)

Week 4: Feel Safe, Strong, and Protected (pages 165–169)

Week 5: Become Genetically Thin (pages 169–170)

Week 6: Improve Your Digestion (pages 171–174)

Week 7: Detox (pages 174–175)

Week 8: Activate the "Get Thin" Programs with Movement (pages 175–176)

Week 9: Reverse Leptin and Insulin Resistance (pages 177)

Week 10: Release Trauma (pages 178–180)

Week 11: Heal Your Body (pages 180–182)

All of these visualizations are in Appendix B, and I've also recorded three of them for you. To access these free bonus audio tracks, please visit www.TheGabrielMethod.com/visualization-bonus.

Reinforce Your Visualizations

Whenever you think of it during the day, reinforce whatever visualization you listened to that morning by doing a quick version of it. For example, if the visualization prompts you to imagine the weight melting off your body, then during the day as you're walking to work, or sitting at your desk, just imagine for a second the same image of the weight melting off your body. If your morning visualization prompts you to imagine a column of light protecting your body, then, whenever you happen to think of it, imagine that column of light covering your body and you feeling safe and protected by it. Literally a second or two is all it takes to reinforce. The reason is, when you create the image during your visualization it becomes like a program that you can activate at will. SMART Mode is the programming mode you are in when you make the visual image. With the program in place, you can recall it anytime you like during the day and still get the same tremendous benefit.

Add Real Foods

As you're going through this process, remember to add as much real food as possible per my suggestions in Chapter 14. The more real food you eat, the more nourished you'll be and the more energy you'll have. You'll also crave less junk food and feel satiated sooner, and this will make the process much easier. Don't turn this into a rigid, restrictive diet, because as we know, that's not sustainable. Just keep the focus on adding—adding, adding, adding—add real, fresh, live, and organic salads, fruits, nuts, seeds, sprouts, fermented and cultured veggies, grass-fed animal protein, and wild-caught fish. Add lots of omega-3s, too. Try to add one real food each day.

Then give yourself plenty of time for the visualizations to kick in. Soon you'll get to a place where all you crave is real food and your body starts to *naturally* reject dead, processed, highly chemical-laden man-made foods. Read labels carefully but know as a general rule, the best labels are *no* labels. A head of lettuce or a filet of wild-caught salmon have no labels or list of ingredients. They just are what they are—perfect the way nature created them.

By the time you finish these 16 weeks, you will have laid the groundwork for permanent, sustainable weight loss. Your mind and body will be working in perfect synchronicity. You'll feel protected and strong, you won't be as hungry, and your body will be letting go of weight. Your brain will be rewired to be resilient to stress, you'll be more socially connected, and you'll have resolved past traumatic issues. Your chemistry will reset so that you're more sensitive to fat-burning hormones. You'll have activated the genetic expression of your thin genes. You'll be attracting success, abundance, and love. Most important, you'll have positive momentum surging through your life and redirecting your future. You'll feel as if you have a new sense of control over the destiny of your life.

The visualization methods in this book are about weight loss, but they're also about so much more. I used visualization to stop migraines, stop smoking, increase my business, and address numerous other issues. This is a creative tool that you can use to improve your overall health and solve any and all of your problems. What's important is to learn the skill, and to practice it daily.

I still practice visualization and meditation every morning, and I find it to be one of the most pleasurable, powerful, enjoyable experiences in my life. It takes me to a place where I'm filled with joy, peace, light, and love and where I feel thoroughly energized with life force energy. My hope is that you'll do the same, and you'll be inspired to practice visualization on a daily basis, joining me and hundreds of thousands of people around the world who have used the Gabriel Method to achieve success.

So I invite you to begin this journey with me by first taking the 16-week visualization for weight loss challenge, and then go on to apply visualization to any and all areas of your life. The results may be so great that you get to the same place that I have: A few years down the road, you'll look at your life and realize that the weight you had to lose—the weight that was once such a painful and frustrating part of your life—has actually become a blessing in disguise. Because in finding a solution to your weight issues, you were introduced to a part of yourself that you didn't even know you had. You've tapped into your creative essence in a way you could not possibly have imagined, and you've used that creative power to transform not only your body but your entire life as well. I'm holding that vision for you . . . Let's hold that vision together and make it happen!

FREQUENTLY ASKED QUESTIONS

Can I listen to visualizations while driving?

No! Please never listen to our visualizations while driving or operating heavy machinery. You need to be able to relax while listening. Also please don't listen to them while someone else who's driving can hear them.

Visualization brings up painful memories or makes me cry. Should I still do it?

Absolutely. Crying is one of the most healing things you can do emotionally. It's your body's way of cleaning out emotional toxins. So if the visualization brings tears to your eyes, if it brings unpleasant memories and you're releasing them through crying, it means that your body's letting go of those emotions, which is exactly what you want to happen.

I fall asleep listening to the evening visualization. Is that okay?

The evening visualization is designed for you to fall asleep listening to it. It's got a frequency-following pattern that puts you into the SMART Mode states of alpha, theta, and then eventually the delta state, and allows your body to drift off into a deep state of sleep. While you're sleeping, your mind will still be very receptive to all the positive suggestions, so you'll still be reaping all the benefits. It's actually a great scenario, because it puts you in a deep state of sleep, while your brain is being prompted to make positive suggestions for healthy lifestyle and eating habits.

My mind wanders. Is that okay?

It's totally okay if your mind wanders. I once heard a quote that 99 percent of success in life was just showing up, and nowhere is that more true than with visualization. You just want to show up, just want to press the button and listen to the visualization. If your mind wanders, it's okay, because over time you'll start getting into deeper and deeper states of clarity and focus, and your mind won't wander. Either way, even if your mind is wandering, you'll still benefit from the suggestions.

I can't concentrate. Is that okay?

That's totally fine. Don't worry if you can't concentrate. As a matter of fact, in the beginning don't even try to concentrate. If you try too hard to concentrate, it's actually going to take you out of the deep state that you want to get into when you're doing your visualization, and it's going to require too much effort and you'll get frustrated and you won't continue. So allow your mind to wander. Don't worry if you can't concentrate. It's totally okay, and over time you'll get better and better. Visualization is like a muscle that gets stronger and stronger with use.

What if I can't imagine my ideal body?

Many people can't imagine their ideal body, and that's okay. There are a couple of things you can do. One is to find a picture of either when you were in your ideal body or a picture of someone else who has a body similar to the one you'd like to create, and right before your visualization just stare at it for about 30 seconds. Then close your eyes and imagine yourself looking like that image. If you can't imagine it, just feel it. Feel what it feels like to have no excess weight on you. Feel what it feels like to be walking on the beach, thin and fit. You can also feel what it feels like to have all the fat melting off your body as you're sitting there. So you don't have to worry if you can't see it. Just try as best as you can to feel it.

I can't imagine light going through any part of my body. Is that okay?

Whatever the suggestions are for the visualizations, don't worry if you can't see them or imagine them. Simply imagine what you can imagine, and the rest of the time just stay present as best you can and allow yourself to get into a relaxed state.

What if I can't sit for too long without feeling uncomfortable?

It's really important for you to do the visualizations in a position that you're comfortable in. So if you can't sit while you're doing the visualizations, then lay down in a comfortable position.

How do I know it's working?

What you'll find, once you've been doing visualizations for a while, is that you'll experience a subtle shift in the way you approach your body weight, food, exercise, and activity. You'll find that you're not as hungry, you don't crave the same fattening foods, your blood sugar stays stable longer, you're simply not thinking about food as much, and you have more energy. You'll also notice a shift in the way you think and feel about your body. You'll start to become more loving, forgiving, accepting, and appreciative of your body. This can happen fairly quickly or it can take a little bit of time, but that's the first indication that there's been a shift in your body's chemistry toward letting go of weight.

How do I know when I'm in SMART Mode?

When you're doing your visualizations, if your mind starts to calm down a little bit and if you find as you're sitting that you're less inclined to fidget or move, then you're beginning to get into the SMART Mode states.

I fidget. Is that okay?

If you're fidgeting in the beginning, don't worry, that's totally fine, but what you will find over time is that your body will start to become calmer and you're going to be less likely to want to fidget or want to move, and eventually you'll get to a place where your mind and your body become very calm and still.

I can't see anything when I visualize. What do I do?

When you're listening to the guided visualizations, don't worry if you can't see anything. Just feel whatever you can feel, imagine whatever you can imagine, and simply be present for the visualization. Over time, it will start working better and better, even if you can't see anything, you're still communicating with your body and you'll still get tremendous benefit.

What if I can't get into SMART Mode?

Getting into the relaxed state of SMART Mode is a natural process that we all go through every night as we're going to sleep, only in this case we're doing it while we're awake. If you can't do it in the beginning, once again, don't worry. It's like a muscle that gets stronger over time and your ability to go into those states becomes quicker and easier. Simply be present and show up for the visualization each day, and eventually you'll be able to get into that state without any effort at all.

When should I visualize?

The best time to visualize is first thing in the morning, as soon as you get up, and also just as you are going to sleep. In the morning, you will be programming your day for success, and at night your mind and subconscious will be processing the positive visual images and suggestions you imagined as you are going to sleep. Ideally, for the morning session, what you want to do is have an area all set up just for your visualization, where all you have to do is sit up and press Play and listen to the visualization as soon as you arise.

If you can't practice visualization first thing in the morning, the second-best choice is simply to aim for consistency. Choose a specific time when you can practice visualization every day, because what will happen is your body will get used to the stress-reduction benefits that come from visualization at a certain time during the day.

For the evening visualization, you simply want to visualize as you are going to sleep. Another great time to practice visualization is in the late afternoons approximately an hour or two before you come home from work or an hour or two before dinner. I call this a stress-reduction break. Have a healthy snack and listen to a visualization, and it will help reduce the stress of the day and keep your blood sugar stable so that when you come home from work, you won't be famished, exhausted, and stressed out, and you'll be better able to make good food and lifestyle choices the rest of the night.

How often should I visualize?

It's important to visualize every day, even if it's just for a couple of minutes. What will happen over time, if you do it every day, is your brain will start making neural connections toward feelings of peace, safety, love, and healthy lifestyle choices and away from the connections of fear and stress, and that will have a tremendous benefit in your life. It takes some time to rewire your brain, but it will happen much quicker if you do it every single day. Also, if you do it every day, it will start to become a habit. Then it takes on a life of its own, and it becomes one of the most beneficial and pleasurable experiences that you can have over time.

How much time should I spend practicing?

There's no limit to how much time you can spend practicing, but at the very least spend a couple of minutes each day. The daytime visualizations that I make are usually less than ten minutes long. But you may find that you want to continue visualizing after the recording is over, because you're feeling calm and relaxed and your body doesn't want to move. So if you feel like it, just stay in that meditative state and visualize some more.

I have a pacemaker. Can I do it?

If you have a pacemaker, you don't want to listen to the visualizations we've created with music, because the music has a frequency-following response built into it, and sometimes that frequency-following response can interfere with the pacemaker. You can check with your doctor. Some doctors say it's fine, some may not, but you can listen to the visualizations without music and you can practice visualizations on your own.

I have epilepsy. Can I do it?

If you have epilepsy, you don't want to listen to the visualizations with music, because the frequency-following response is similar to a strobe light and can cause a seizure. But check with your doctor; he or she may say it's fine for you. Either way, it's totally fine to listen to the visualizations without music and to practice visualizations on your own.

After I've reached my goal, what visualization should I listen to?

After you've reached your goal, you can listen to any visualization you want. It doesn't matter. Or you can start practicing visualizations on your own. Instead of listening to the visualization first thing in the morning, just sit up and do your own visualization in the morning and let that start to take on a positive momentum and develop a life of its own.

I've been listening to the visualization but have not lost any weight. Why?

Sometimes it can take time to address the real issues and to change your body hormonally and chemically. I've had people lose tremendous amounts of weight, but it took them several months before it started. If you're noticing changes in your body where you're less hungry and you have more energy and you're craving healthier foods, that's a clear indication that there are changes taking place, but it still may take time. So be patient and continue, and what you may find is you'll get to a certain place where all of a sudden you start losing weight.

When will I start losing weight after listening to visualizations?

There's no one-size-fits-all answer to that question. Some people lose weight quickly, as soon as they start practicing visualization. For other people, it can take months before any weight loss appears. But you will notice differences when you start visualizing that are indications that changes are taking place, such as having more energy, craving less junk food, craving healthier foods, and going longer periods of time without being hungry. These are all indications that hormonal changes are taking place in your body, and it's just a question of time as to when the weight loss will start. So if it doesn't happen immediately, definitely persevere.

Which visualization should I do?

You can listen to any visualization you want. There's no wrong way to visualize. You can never listen to a wrong visualization. If you're attracted to a certain visualization because it makes you feel good or because it touches something in you, then that's a good visualization to listen to. If you've got specific life issues that you want to work on, such as improving your abundance, healing your digestion, keeping your blood sugar stable, reducing stress, strengthening your boundaries, or working through emotional issues, then you can listen to those specific visualizations. Otherwise, any visualization you listen to will yield benefits.

If I'm going through a painful divorce or other life-changing situation, how can I use visualization to help me?

If you're going through a challenging divorce or breakup or changing jobs, the best thing you can do is visualize everything working out incredibly well, during your visualizations and also during the day. Instead of holding on to the fear and uncertainty, visualize your most ideal scenario, separating from your spouse in a healthy, happy way, having it be amicable, having the family be happy, maybe being with somebody else if that's appropriate, and having that scenario be beautiful. If you're going through a change with your job, visualize the new job working out tremendously well and having it be everything you expected. Stay focused on the positive, and use visualization to imagine your most ideal scenario throughout the day, and it will help direct you and attract for you the most ideal scenario.

GUIDED VISUALIZATIONS FOR THE 16-WEEK TOTAL TRANSFORMATION VISUALIZATION CHALLENGE

These visualizations are actual transcripts of some of my most effective live visualizations. I find that group visualizations are extremely powerful. When I practice in a group I do not script the visualizations, I just set an intention for what the theme of the visualization will be, get into a deep meditative state, and then I simply describe what I see.

You'll find that some of the wording might seem redundant and the tone overly conversational, but I've left them so intentionally to keep the text as true to the actual visualization as possible. The redundancy can be extremely effective in reinforcing positive suggestions.

You can record these visualizations yourself if you like for your own practice or simply take the gist of the visualization and practice it on your own. Or listen to the three recordings I've made. You can also get tremendous benefit by simply reading the visualizations to yourself or someone else. Throughout the text you'll see a series of periods in a row like this ". . .". When you see those marks just break from reading for a few seconds.

The first couple of paragraphs of each visualization are always similar as they are all subtle variations on the Ocean of Energy and Spinning the Spine techniques for getting into SMART Mode.

For this reason I've deleted them from the transcripts. We talk about these techniques for getting into SMART Mode in Chapters 2 and 11. Here they are again for your review. Simply choose either one of them (unless I specify which one to use) and spend a couple of minutes getting into SMART Mode in the beginning of each visualization.

(Note: I've recorded three of these visualizations for you. To access these audio tracks for free, please visit www.TheGabriel Method.com/visualization-bonus.)

VISUALIZATIONS FOR GETTING INTO SMART MODE

Technique 1: Spinning the Spine (Reproduced from Chapter 11)

Imagine a glowing ball of white light, about the size of a golf ball, starting at your navel, then going down to the base of the spine and spinning around each vertebra, one at a time. You have 24 vertebrae in your spine. Don't worry about exactly where each vertebra is; just imagine the ball of light spinning around the base of your spine a few times and then going up one notch at a time, 24 times. After you've gone up about five notches, you should imagine the ball of light to be around the middle of your stomach, then after about 12 to 14 vertebrae, behind your heart. When it gets to 17, you're in your neck, and when you get to 24 you're at the base your skull. Then imagine the ball of light going into your head, then your face, front of your neck, your heart, and then again into your stomach. By the time the ball gets back to your stomach, you should be in SMART Mode.

Technique 2: The Ocean of Energy (an expanded version of the technique we discussed in Chapter 2)

When you're ready, just sit up straight, take a deep breath in and take a deep breath out, and relax. Imagine that there's a bright ball of bright white light circulating around your navel. Maybe it's the size of a large softball or a volleyball. And it's just circulating around your navel like a spiral or vortex of a galaxy of light. Just beautiful, bright, healing white light. And as it's circulating around your navel, it's getting brighter and brighter. And as this beautiful, bright ball of white light is circulating around your navel, I'd like you to also imagine that you're in an infinite ocean of beautiful, bright, healing white light.

It's an infinite ocean as far as you can possibly see in all directions of bright white healing light. And this light has the power to heal your body.

And I'd just like you to imagine that as you're sitting there in this ocean of bright white light, that the pores of your skin open up, and this bright white healing light comes rushing into your body from all directions. It's covering your body, energizing your body, and filling your body with bright white light. You can feel bright white light rushing into your torso, your chest, your neck, your head, and your arms and legs. You can feel this bright white healing light rushing into the bones of your body, filling your bones with bright white vibrant life force energy. So the bones in your arms and in your legs and all over your body, all of your bones, are glowing with bright white light. And your muscles are glowing with bright white light, and your organs are being filled with bright, healing, energizing light. Imagine the ocean of energy filling your chest and your lungs with light, feel it going into your stomach and digestive tract. See the energy filling your liver, kidneys, spleen, pancreas, gall bladder, and your entire torso with bright white healing light.

Now imagine the energy going into your heart and filling your heart with healing bright white light. And as your heart is filled with bright white light, it energizes the blood that passes through your heart. So supercharged bright glowing blood is circulating through your body now, from your left side to your right, filling every cell of your body with a luminous, glowing, healing energy. And you can now imagine every cell of your body glowing, with beautiful bright white healing energy.

Now as you're sitting there with your entire body glowing with energy and this ball of bright white light in your navel, imagine that any excess weight you have becomes white light and gets sucked into the center of your navel, into the center of the vortex never to be seen again. So any excess weight on your thighs or your stomach or your chest or your arms or your face is all being sucked into this whirlpool, this vortex in your navel.

And as that's happening and as you're sitting there, you're starting to realize that you're in your most perfect, ideal shape. Any excess weight that you've had has now been sucked into this vortex never to be seen again, and you're sitting there and you're in your most perfect, ideal shape. You can feel your stomach firm, flat, and tight; your legs light and strong; and your whole body glowing with health, fitness, and vitality.

Now that every cell of your body is glowing with energy, you are now ready to continue with your desired visualization.

WEEK 1: BELIEVE YOUR BODY WANTS TO BE THIN

NOTE—Use either the Ocean of Light or Spinning the Spine visualization to get into SMART Mode. End this part of the visualization imagining a ball of bright white light circulating around your navel . . .

And as that ball of energy is spinning around your navel, I'd like you to imagine that it becomes like a whirlpool or a vortex and it starts pulling energy into it . . .

Imagine that all the excess weight on your body has become liquid energy. It's no longer physical; it's just energy. So imagine any excess weight on your body has become like a liquid energy that's being sucked into this whirlpool never to be seen again . . . So any excess weight on your thighs or your stomach or your chest or your arms or your face is all being sucked into this whirlpool, this vortex in your navel.

And as that's happening and as you're sitting there, you're start-ing to realize that you're in your most perfect, ideal shape . . . Any excess weight that you've had has now been sucked into this vortex never to be seen again, and you're sitting there in your most perfect, ideal shape.

Just feel what that feels like for a minute, to be in your most perfect, ideal shape . . .

Now imagine that as you're sitting there in your most perfect, ideal shape, you stand up (in your mind's eye) and you're walking on the beach . . .

. . . It's a beautiful sunny day and you're in your most perfect, ideal shape; the sun is out and you're walking and the water is caressing your ankles and you can feel the cool water on your feet and the warm sun on your shoulders.

Maybe as you're walking in your most perfect, ideal shape, you put some sun lotion on your skin and you feel how tight your stomach is, and your arms and your body, and you're feeling light and you're moving really quickly and easily . . .

Now imagine that as you're walking, you start to move fast-er and faster and faster, and pretty soon for no reason at all you just start running just because you can and just because it feels so amazing . . .

And you can feel that you're in your most perfect, ideal shape, and you're running out of just pure joy and energy and passion . . .

Remember this is a visualization . . . and you can have whatev-er you imagine, so simply just imagine that you're running, glid-ing, skipping effortlessly like the wind . . .

You're just imagining that you're in your most perfect, ideal shape and you're running on the beach, and you're kicking the water as you run, and after a while maybe you turn and face the water and you jump over one wave and then a second wave; then you dive into the water just because it feels so good, and you feel the cool refreshing water on your skin.

Then imagine that you jump up in the air and you raise your hands just out of pure joy, and you say, "This is me. This is my ideal shape. This is who I am. My body wants to be like this; my body wants to be fit!" And you're feeling that in every cell, at every level of your being that this is your most perfect, ideal self, and you're creating that for yourself now.

Then bringing your attention back to your body, as you're sitting there now back in this room, you can sort of still feel the sun that was on your skin . . .

You can feel that you're in your perfect, ideal shape.

You feel a little bit tighter and stronger.

And now I'd just like you to imagine the rest of your day, and I'd like you to imagine how the rest of your day you're being filled with energy and vitality and passion and inspiration and how incredibly well it's going for you, and you're making new friends and the sun is shining and the food is delicious and you're feeling beautiful and healthy and happy and understanding your body and your mind, and knowing that your body now wants to be thin.

Imagine, how the next couple of days go, where as each day goes you're feeling healthier and happier and fitter . . . and maybe you're not as hungry and maybe have just a little bit more spring in your step. And people are looking at you and they're saying, "Wow, you look amazing . . . You look so different . . . Something is different about you."

You're calmer . . . and you're more centered . . . and you're more focused . . . and people are so engaged by you. You've got a powerful magnetic presence and people are riveted when you're talking to them . . . Maybe you're in a sales meeting or maybe you're meeting with clients . . . and they're totally captivated by your energy and your power and your presence.

Maybe it's midday and you've got lots of energy, you're not tired, you're not exhausted.

You're craving healthier foods and positive things are flowing in your family and your relationships and you're feeling safer and more centered.

And as each day goes by, you're losing weight, you're feeling fitter, more successful, having more energy, more light, and more vitality, and your energy is bursting with light. And you can imagine how in six months from now everything in your life has changed.

You've lost the weight that you need to lose and it's effortless and you're on an incredible high and there's momentum in your life.

And now you can imagine how a year from now, and two years from now, how everything's changed because you now have health and energy and vitality and calmness and passion and inspiration and you're effortlessly fit and you feel safe and supported by everyone and everything in your life.

And in your own time and space, when you're ready, just open your eyes and know that you've just planted a seed so that forever your life will be changed positively and forever you'll be thinner, fitter, more positive, more successful, happier, and have a more joyous life, and you will lose weight easily, naturally, and effortlessly, because your body now wants to be thin.

WEEK 2: NOURISH YOUR BODY

NOTE—Use the Ocean of Energy visualization to get into SMART Mode. End this part of the visualization imagining a ball of bright white light circulating around your navel and your body in an infinite ocean of energy . . .

And as every cell in your body is charged with this superbright white healing light, you can imagine that every cell of your body is saying at the same time the words . . . "Nourished, nourished, nourished, I feel nourished, nourished, nourished. I feel complete, whole, satisfied, alive, healthy, fit, vibrant." Just every cell of your body . . . 70 trillion cells in your body, saying at the same time like a chorus, "Nourished, nourished, nourished, nourished. I feel alive. I feel vibrant. I feel satisfied. I feel whole, complete, loved, supported."

And as every cell in your body feels nourished, you can imagine now that any excess weight on your body just disappears. It just gets washed away into this ocean of white light, never to be seen again. And you're sitting there in your most perfect, ideal weight, in your most perfect, ideal body, feeling whole, complete, nourished, supported, protected, loved . . . And you can imagine yourself walking down the street later today or maybe tomorrow, and feeling the same feeling of being totally nourished and energized . . . glowing with a beautiful bright white light . . . So much energy . . . And you can imagine yourself walking on the street in your most perfect, ideal shape, feeling totally energized, satisfied, loved, nourished, supported, totally complete.

And maybe you pass a bakery or some other shop that you might normally stop in to get a quick hit of energy, and you just look at it and you smile and you think to yourself, "I don't need that. I have so much energy right now." You're glowing with energy. You're like your own sun, totally glowing with energy. You don't need the energy. You don't need the short-term, addictive fix of junk food anymore. You have energy, and you are so nourished. And you can see yourself day after day, getting fitter, healthier, happier, feeling more loved, more supported, more nourished . . .

And you can also imagine how this beautiful bright white light is nourishing your head and your mind. Every brain cell and every particle of your consciousness is just being bathed in this beautiful white healing light, and you feel calm, centered, secure, powerful, relaxed, totally satisfied, and totally nourished . . .

And you can imagine yourself now during the day, what your day is going to be like. Maybe you'll be at the office, maybe you'll be with friends or family or kids, and you can see yourself feeling calm and radiant and relaxed, feeling safe, strong, protected, nourished, loved, supported, energized . . . You don't need the excess weight anymore . . . You don't crave those foods anymore, just because you feel so totally energized, so totally supported. It's like the universe has just plugged you into an infinite stream of energy, and you feel always supported and you're radiating divine light; your very bones are glowing with this beautiful bright white healing light, and life is effortless. Life is so easy, and there's so much flow . . .

You're vibrating at a higher frequency. And so you're having higher-frequency experiences. And when you are hungry, you're craving higher-frequency foods. So you can see yourself throughout your day, when you do eat, eating, real, live, super-high-vitality foods . . . Foods that are glowing with life force vitality. And when you eat them you feel truly nourished, sustained, and supported. You can see yourself eating and craving real, live, high-vitality foods, loving them, having a bite or two and feeling your entire body be instantly nourished and instantly satisfied. Dead foods seem coarse and impure to you, and your body now naturally rejects them and favors real, live, high-vitality foods. And as you eat these foods you're being charged with life force vitality. See how the food travels through your body, filling your every cell with nourishment, vitality, and life force energy. See your energy radiating and flowing through your body as you get brighter and healthier . . .

Your energy is flowing and so your life is flowing. You can see how your life is flowing day after day, as you're getting fitter and healthier and happier. You're losing weight effortlessly and easily, and you're feeling calm, centered, supported, radiant, totally nourished, totally energized, and in every way possible feeling like life and your body and your mind are pure, divine, perfection.

And in your own time and space, when you're ready, you can open your eyes, knowing that you have just plugged into an infinite source of energy that's nourishing you. It's nourishing your body. It's nourishing your mind. It's nourishing your being. It's nourishing you at every level. And because it's nourishing you, you don't need the weight anymore, and you're calm, centered, protected, and secured. And every day you lose weight and get fitter effortlessly, until you have reached your ideal weight . . .

And in your own time and space, when you're ready, you can open your eyes.

WEEK 3: REDUCE STRESS

NOTE—Use either the Ocean of Light or Spinning the Spine visualization to get into SMART Mode. End this part of the visualization imagining a ball of bright white light circulating around your navel . . .

Imagine your whole body now is just a liquid energy, and you've got this ball of light circulating around your navel—and it's spinning like a vortex or a whirlpool, and any extra weight you have on your body is also like a liquid light, and that liquid light, that excess weight, is being sucked into the vortex in your navel, so that any extra weight you have is being transformed into liquid energy. It's being sucked into your navel, where it can be stored invisibly as liquid energy, whenever you need it.

And so you're sitting there in your most perfect, ideal shape, all the excess weight is gone, it's all been sucked into your navel never to be seen again, only to be used as liquid energy when you need it, invisible life force energy . . . You've transformed the fat in your body into invisible life force energy that you can use whenever you need energy . . .

And you're sitting there in your most perfect, ideal shape, and you're calm and you're centered and you're secure and you're confident and you're fit and your entire body is glowing with a beautiful bright white life force energy.

And as you're sitting there in your most perfect, ideal shape, I'd like you to imagine what the rest of your day is going to be. Whether you're going to be at an office or home, or out with friends and family, I'd like you to imagine your day flowing smoothly, easily, and successfully. Imagine this ocean of energy is always around you, filling your body with life force energy and making you feel calm and relaxed . . .

People are moving around and everyone is as busy as always and you're incredibly productive, but you're also calm and relaxed and people are noticing it. And it's almost like people are gravitating to you because of your calmness. They're all moving around, they're unsure, they might be stressed out, but you're calm, you're relaxed, and you can even see that you're actually glowing with a bright, beautiful life force energy that helps you be extremely focused and extremely creative.

So as people are coming up to you at work perhaps, you can easily solve their problems—whatever the issue is, you find a creative approach instantly, easily, effortlessly. You find a creative approach to whatever the problem is, and nothing can bother you because you feel so confident, so relaxed . . . and you feel so confident and so relaxed because you've got this powerful, bright life force energy protecting you and guiding you and nourishing you and helping you find extremely creative solutions in all situations. You're under control, you're relaxed and confident and radiating health, beauty, confidence, and life force vitality . . .

So you might be in a business meeting, and you're easily asserting whatever is the point that you might want to make, and people are listening and they're almost spellbound by your energy and your confidence. They want to do business with you because they feel so amazing around you. You just feel so calm, and people want that. People want to be around you, because you are calm and confident and centered, and the day goes by easily and effortlessly. You have so much energy.

When it's time to eat, you eat relaxed. There's no hurry. And you can see yourself choosing vibrant, healthy, nutritious, and delicious foods, eating them slowly . . . And as the day goes by, at the end of the day, you're calm and you walk out of work, slowly, relaxed. There's no hurry . . . You're not hungry . . . You're still glowing with life force energy . . .

Imagine the day going incredibly successfully—so much more successfully than you could have ever thought possible . . . and it just seems like, now that you're glowing with life force energy, that opportunities just come to you. It's like you're a flame, and opportunities are drawn to the flame like moths drawn to a fire . . . Opportunities just come to you effortlessly, because you have life force energy glowing through your body.

And so work is incredibly successful and effortlessly successful, successful beyond your wildest imaginations. And you can
imagine six months from now, how you're doing so much better
at work than you ever possibly imagined. You're selling so much
more, you're producing so much more, you're healing so much
more, you're teaching so much more. Whatever it is that you're
doing, it's so much more powerful than you ever could have possibly imagined. You can see yourself glowing and confident . . .
You've built up this positive spiral momentum, where the more
successful you are, the more energy you have, the more people
want to do business with you, and it keeps growing and growing
and growing and growing, and all the while you are relaxed and
effortlessly creative and successful . . .

And you can imagine yourself coming home at the end of
the day and you're meeting your family or your friends or just
relaxing. And you're feeling wonderful, so much energy. It's almost like you didn't go to work at all, or it's almost like the work
energized you because it was so successful and so creative and so
relaxing and so enjoyable. And so at the end of the day you're
not tired. You have energy to go for a walk or a swim or go to the
beach or play with your kids, go out to dinner with your loved
one or your friends and family . . . You've got energy throughout
the day, life force energy, and you can even see yourself glowing with this life force energy from the beginning of the day to
the end of the day, every single day, and you know now that life
will never be the same because you've awakened this incredible,
powerful, relaxing, healing, and creative life force that's coursing
through your veins, and you're living a different life now . . . Successful, fit, confident, healthy, happy, creative beyond your wildest
imagination, and calm, confident.

And so in your own time and space, when you're ready, you
can open your eyes, knowing that you have forever changed your
life for the better and that your life will forever be incredibly
successful, powerful, and fulfilling, for you and everyone in your
life, and that you will continue to get healthier, fitter, happier, and

more successful in every way possible . . . So in your own time and space, please open your eyes.

WEEK 4: FEEL SAFE, STRONG, AND PROTECTED

NOTE—Use either the Ocean of Light or Spinning the Spine visualization to get into SMART Mode. End this part of the visualization imagining a ball of bright white light circulating around your navel . . .

Now imagine a column of light coming down from the sky and surrounding your body. Just a large column of light about arm's length wide, coming from the infinite sky, surrounding your body and going deep into the earth . . . As this column of light surrounds your body, it protects you and supports you and fills your body with bright white healing light. And this column is totally impenetrable. Nothing could possibly touch you that you didn't want to touch you as long as this column of light is around you. Just to demonstrate how powerful this column of light is, imagine it in the distance on some train tracks. A train could smash into this column of light and it could never even touch you. You wouldn't even feel the slightest tremor.

You can even imagine it. You can see this column of light on train tracks in the distance. The train has no passengers. You can see the train smash into the column of light and the train rolls off the tracks. The column of light is totally unaffected. It doesn't even budge . . .

So this incredibly, unbelievably powerful, impenetrable column of light is coming from the sky, and it's wrapping around you, going deep into the center of the earth. And as it wraps around you, it protects you, nourishes you, and supports you. It fills your body up with light and it feels really good. Your whole body is glowing with this protective white light. And you can feel that column of white light, you can touch it with your hands if you want. You can even put your hand through it if you wanted to, and then bring it back out. Imagine yourself touching the sides of the column of light, putting your hand through it and then bringing it back.

And then if you're willing, I'd like you to also imagine there is a big, beautiful bright white angel 12 feet high coming down from the sky. It's a bright, beautiful, extremely powerful guardian angel. And he or she is wrapping his or her wings around you and wrapping his or her wings around the column of light . . .

So you've got this impenetrable column of light that nobody can touch. No thought, no words, no action—nothing—nobody can touch. And then you've got this bright, beautiful, enormously powerful angel wrapping its wings around that column of light and around you, supporting you and protecting you and nourishing you and loving you and going with you wherever you go throughout your day . . .

And as you're in this column of light and these angel wings are around you supporting you and protecting you, I'd like you to imagine that any excess weight on your body just melts off you and goes into the ground. It just becomes part of the white light and just falls into the earth. So you're sitting there or standing there (in your mind's eye) and you're in your most perfect, ideal weight, most perfect, ideal shape. And you're totally safe and totally relaxed and totally calm and totally protected and totally nourished and loved and supported and energized . . . Loved, energized, supported, protected, and calm. You're feeling safe. Safe to let go of the excess weight and safe to live in your most perfect, ideal body and to live your most perfect, ideal life.

And you can imagine walking through your day, maybe tomorrow or the next day when you go home . . . you're walking down the street and you're in your most perfect, ideal shape feeling totally fit, totally happy, and totally protected. And wherever you go, this powerful, bright, supportive, nurturing, impenetrable column of light is with you, surrounding and protecting you . . . And this bright, beautiful, enormously powerful guardian angel is wrapping its wings around you, energizing you, nourishing you, supporting you, and protecting you . . .

And maybe you go to the office, and what you notice is that there's no stress because you just feel safe and protected. People might be upset and you're smiling at them. You're calm and protected and supported and thin and fit. And as you're smiling at them, even though they might be upset, they start to smile back and things start to flow . . .

And maybe you're at a meeting and you're relaxed and calm and protected and projecting this powerful, beautiful white love energy out at the meeting, and people are spellbound . . . they're mesmerized by you. And whatever it is that you're speaking about— they're so interested, and it's received so well and you're successful. And the meeting is successful and the workday's successful and you're energized, happy, calm, content, and at peace . . .

And maybe can imagine going home . . . you're in the house with the people you love and you're feeling safe and calm and protected and nurtured and you're able to nurture them and they're just feeling incredible around you. Everyone's safe, protected, nurtured. There's no conflict because there's such an incredible, beautiful radiance coming out of you that anyone that's anywhere near you can feel. So everyone feels happy, safe, nourished, protected, loved, secure, and loving toward you . . .

It's contagious. It's a vibration. You're projecting the energy of love, safety, happiness, health, contentment, success, and it's contagious . . . People start vibrating at your frequency. So your children are happy, healthy, successful, safe, protected. Your spouse is loving, supportive, happy, protected. Your parents, if they're around, are in the room, too, and they're feeling happy, supportive, and loving . . . They know how amazing you are and they can't help but feel it . . . And there's no limit to how much love and happiness and safety and support that's emanating from you. It's infinite and it's endless. And those angel wings are supporting you and that column of light is there and you're in this ball of energy that's just radiating love and protection.

And anybody else that's important to you or anyone else you might have a challenging relationship with—imagine them in the room with you and you feeling calm, safe, supported, and protected . . . maybe imagine how they might have been uncomfortable to start with, but now they're smiling, they're accepting, they're happy, they're loving. They actually want to hug you and you can actually let them hug you because nothing can hurt you, no negative energy. And you're relaxed and you're just emanating love . . .

And all the excess weight is gone. You don't need it anymore. You have an extra spring in your step as you're walking down the street. You can run as fast as you want and those angel wings will be there all the time. This column of light will be there all the time. They're always with you. You don't need the weight anymore. You don't need it anymore and it's gone. You allow it to just simply melt into the earth . . .

You've got energy, you've got protection, you've got safety and security, and you've got love and nourishment and support . . . Support is all around you. Every cell of your body is being bathed in support. The earth is supporting you. The column of light is supporting you. The angel wings are wrapped around you, loving you, supporting you, adoring you, protecting you, and nurturing you. You are the essence of love and you just allow that to be . . .

And all the stress, tension, fear, or worry that you've ever had all melts away. It's all gone now. You have everything you need now, and life will just get more successful and more prosperous . . .

You're vibrating at a higher frequency and so you're living a higher-frequency life, which means you have higher-frequency experiences—experiences of joy, of success, of abundance, of fitness, of flow, of happiness, of super love, and of joy and peace. Because you're vibrating at such a high frequency, no harm could ever touch you. Harm is at a much lower frequency. You're at a much higher frequency. You're 100 stories above any type of harm. You're floating in protection and love.

And once more, coming back into the room, feeling that ball of energy in your stomach and the energy coming out from the earth and the energy coming down from the sky, and the column of light that's wrapped around you and the angel wings that are wrapped around you . . .

In your own time and space, when you're ready, you can open your eyes and know that you are forever loved and support- ed and protected, and the weight will now simply dissolve. And when you know that to be true, in your own time and space, and when you feel better, and you can feel it now, you can just simply open your eyes.

WEEK 5: BECOME GENETICALLY THIN

NOTE—Use the Ocean of Energy visualization to get into SMART Mode. End this part of the visualization imagining a ball of bright white light circulating around your navel and your body in an infinite ocean of energy . . .

I'd like you to imagine again that any excess weight you have becomes just a liquid light that gets sucked into this ball of light in your navel, never to be seen again.

Very quickly now this time, all the excess weight, like in a sec- ond, gets sucked into this navel. And you're sitting there in your most perfect, ideal shape.

And as you're sitting there in your most perfect, ideal shape, I'd like you to imagine again that you're going for a walk on the beach and you see yourself walking and you're fit and you're healthy and you're happy and you're vibrant.

It's a beautiful sunny day—take this image of you being fit and healthy and happy and imagine this image goes into one of the cells of your body, like a little mini-image of you, perfectly fit, healthy, happy, ideal, in your most ideal shape, is in one of the cells of your body, a little mini-version of you.

It actually goes into the DNA in your cells.

It's standing next to one of the strands of the DNA in your cells, and it walks over to the DNA and it moves into it, and the second it does you feel your DNA vibrate like a string and with this vibration your DNA has just changed . . . You've just repro- grammed yourself on a genetic level to be genetically thin. You've just changed the genetic structure of that cell, so that that cell is now genetically thin, your exact, perfect, ideal body . . . That DNA has just been changed . . .

And now just imagine in an instant, every single cell in your body changes exactly the same, like a wave, it spreads from one cell to the next . . . In an instant, every cell has changed, so that you've just reprogrammed yourself on a cellular level, at the level of your DNA, to be genetically thin.

Feeling that change—knowing that something has just changed on a genetic level, that somehow genetically, at the level of the DNA, you have changed ever so slightly so that your body now wants to be thin, and so weight loss is effortless, easy, and natural.

You can imagine now the rest of the day, feeling healthy, fit, vibrant, energetic, full, and content . . . Not wanting anywhere near as much food, because your body is now effortlessly burning fat . . . And you can imagine the coming weeks and months, how your body starts to morph into that naturally thin person you've just programmed yourself to be . . .

It's automatic now, it's just a matter of time . . . six weeks, six months down the road, one year, you can see yourself getting fitter and fitter and feeling energetic, successful, healthy, vibrant, and full of life. It's all happening now automatically, now that you're a naturally thin . . . effortlessly thin . . . genetically thin person.

And in your own time, open your eyes and know forever that your body has just been changed on a genetic level and you are now a naturally thin, effortlessly thin person.

WEEK 6: IMPROVE YOUR DIGESTION

I'd like you to imagine a ball of white light circulating around your navel and this ball of white light is getting brighter and brighter and brighter . . .

It's like a galaxy of ultrabright light in your navel and that bright light is energizing your stomach and revitalizing your stomach and purifying your stomach and detoxifying your stomach . . .

And then just imagine that that same bright light that's inside your navel is also outside your body and you are actually in an ocean of bright white light and that light is all around you . . .

The bright light touches your skin and it enters your body and it purifies your skin and energizes your bones. And as that bright light then enters your body, it enters your digestive tract . . .

It enters your mouth . . . your esophagus . . . your stomach . . . your small intestines . . . and your large intestine . . . from one end to the other.

That ocean of bright white vitality energy is entering your digestive tract, it's purifying your digestive tract, it is cleaning out the toxins in your digestive tract, and it's purifying your digestive tract . . .

You've got this ball of white light that is spinning around your navel and I'd like you to imagine that all the excess weight in your body just dissolves into this energy . . .

It becomes an energy itself and rather than being fat it gets transmuted into a different type of energy . . . It gets transmuted into bright white liquid light that gets sucked into your navel, so all the excess weight in your body has gone and you are sitting there in your most perfect, ideal shape without an ounce of excess fat and you feel amazing . . .

Your whole digestive tract from your mouth down to your bottom, your whole digestive tract is glowing with bright white light and vibrance . . .

It's being purified and any of the waste that hasn't been eliminated turns into an energy and gets sucked into the center of your navel and never gets seen again . . . It gets evaporated . . . It gets washed clean so that you've got a brand-new digestive tract. Your whole digestive tract is brand new, all the impurities are eliminated and you are able to digest and assimilate nutrients much better.

So just image as you are sitting there in your most perfect, ideal shape with your digestive tract glowing with bright white light and being regenerated and purified and healed . . .

Then, in your mind's eye, I'd like you to imagine that you stand up and you are walking through your day, and as you are walking through your day you can see your digestive tract from one end to the other glowing with bright white light . . .

You can see yourself healthy, fit, vibrant, and energetic, and you can see yourself in your most perfect, ideal shape so there is not an ounce of excess weight on you . . .

Your digestive tract is totally purified and as you go through your day you can see the foods that you are attracted to; you are attracted to healthy, light, vibrant, rich, colorful, live, beautiful foods . . .

You can see yourself sitting down; there's a beautiful live, vibrant salad with sprouts, and it is glowing with bright white light and any other foods that you might want there . . .

And you're sitting and you're calm and centered and happy as you are about to have a meal and you take a bite of the food . . .

You hold it in your mouth and you chew your food slowly and you feel the energy of this ocean of white light going into the food and energizing it and digesting the food . . .

You see the food that is going into your digestive tract is glowing with white light and easily digested and transformed into energy, and that energy is going into your body and energizing you. You just have a little bit and you're already feeling satisfied . . .

Magically you are feeling satisfied and energized. You can feel the food nourishing your body. It's easily going through your digestion, it is getting into the cells of your body and the cells of your body are glowing with a bright white live vibrance . . .

You are eating live foods and your body is alive again and you feel safe and protected and energized and nourished from this live food and you have lots of energy and you get up and you go through your day and you are glowing; you are actually glowing.

You've got so much life force in your body and you are able to easily go through your work. It's so easy and so effortless and you are fit and light and healthy . . .

And you see yourself in the morning now taking your probiotics and you see yourself eating your digestive enzymes with meals and eating lots of healthy, live salads and your life is flowing, your day is flowing; you have energy, power, amazing stamina and it's just effortless . . .

Everything is so effortless you don't need that much food anymore. You need a couple of bites of food, of real choice, live food and you are energized; your system kicks in and you can see your digestive tract glowing wherever you are . . .

You are at the office, you are with your family, you are playing sports, whatever you are doing. Your digestive tract is purified, glowing, live, vibrant, and healthy and renewed . . .

Your lifeline, your tube to life, your connection to life itself is renewed and energized and is now nourishing and your cells are glowing with bright white light and you have energy to finish your day and the weight is melting off you . . .

You don't need the weight anymore, your body is nourished, it's energized and it's totally protected and so the weight falls off . . . and you only have desires now for the healthiest live food because you are getting energy all the time . . .

You don't need that much energy from food, you are not dependent on dead foods anymore, they actually have no attraction anymore. What attracts you are live, healthy, beautiful, vibrant foods. They energize your body and you feel totally nourished.

Your day flows beautifully, successfully, happily and each day you are getting better and healthier and fitter and thinner and more amazing and more fantastic and more powerful and in every way possible you are living the life of your dreams . . .

And so in your own time and space when you are ready, you can open your eyes knowing that your digestive system is revitalized so that you'll have amazing energy, be attracted to real, live, healthy foods and lose weight easily and effortlessly, now and always.

WEEK 7: DETOX

NOTE—Use the Ocean of Energy visualization to get into SMART Mode. End this part of the visualization imagining a ball of bright white light circulating around your navel and your body in an infinite ocean of energy . . .

And this bright white light goes into your mouth and into your stomach and it clears out any debris in your stomach, just vaporizes it into bright white light . . . And into your intestines . . . Any accumulated waste there is all being vaporized into bright white light. And into your colon and into your anus, it's all being vaporized. Your whole intestinal tract, from your mouth down to your bottom is one glowing, bright white light of vibrancy. Any accumulated waste has been vaporized . . . you've got the most pure digestive tract now, able to easily digest and assimilate nutrients and remove any blockages.

And this bright white light goes into your hips and removes any accumulated waste in your hip joints and your knees and your bones and your ankles and your feet. All the joints of your body . . . it removes any waste, and you're just sitting there in this infinite ocean of energy, this bright white energy, and you are just as bright; you are glowing with bright white light, inside and out . . . Everything is just one bright ball of energy.

And you can imagine this energy start to accumulate and swirl in your navel, like a mini-galaxy. It's swirling around your navel. You've got this ball of bright white energy swirling around your navel, and your whole body is energy. Your whole body is glowing . . . And I'd like you to imagine that any excess weight that you have on your body is also just a glowing, bright light, and it's being sucked into this vortex or this galaxy, this spinning ball of energy in your navel . . .

And so you're sitting there in your most perfect, ideal shape, all the excess weight has been sucked into your navel, and you're glowing with bright white light . . . You've been transmuted into pure, light, liquid energy . . . There's no blockages. There's no accumulated waste. And you can see yourself craving healthy, vibrant foods . . . foods that nourish, heal, and cleanse your body and your body is flushing out all the toxins . . . You can see yourself drinking lots of healthy green juices and water and eating live vibrant foods that are all cleaning your body, purifying it, healing it, and flushing out any accumulated waste . . . And you're getting healthier, cleaner, purer, and fitter, day after day . . .

And wherever you go, you feel this infinite ocean of energy energizing you, running through the pores of your skin, purifying your body, detoxifying your body, and giving you energy all day long . . . You don't need much food anymore, because you have so much energy and vibrance . . . And when you are hungry you crave healthy, live, vibrant foods . . . foods that energize you, nourish you, and purify and cleanse your body. You can see yourself day by day getting healthier, fitter, and purer . . . It's like you've been plugged into a whole different energy system now. And so the weight is melting off you day by day, and you can see yourself glowing with life force vitality—so fit, so pure, and so healthy . . . and you can see the weight melting off you, each day getting thinner, fitter, healthier, more prosperous, happier, more vibrant, cleaner, fitter—craving healthy, live, vibrant foods and feeling amazing . . .

And in your own time and space, when you're ready, you can open your eyes . . .

WEEK 8: ACTIVATE THE "GET THIN" PROGRAMS WITH MOVEMENT

Now imagine that as you're sitting there, you stand up and you go for a walk on the beach. And you have so much energy that you just start walking faster and faster and faster. And there's no excess weight on your body, so you're light and you're fit and you're strong and you're healthy and you're nourished and you're confident and you're secure. And you feel so light that you start walking and actually skipping and even running, and you start running really fast. You can't help it because you're just so light and full of energy now and it's such an amazing feeling that you just can't help but run really fast. So you start running on the beach and you're kicking up water as you run and it's effortless and you're smiling.

And as you're running on the beach, you notice that behind you something is chasing you. It doesn't matter what it is, but you smile because you know that no matter what it is, you can easily outrun it. And you sprint like you have never sprinted in your life. And you smile as you sprint, because you're running so fast and it's so effortless and you're so light and strong and fit, and you can feel as you're running that there's no excess weight on your body. And it feels amazing. You're like an Olympic sprinter. There's no excess weight and you're moving like the wind, and you look back and you easily outrun whatever it is that was chasing you and you smile. And it gave up a long time ago, and you just start walking. And you feel amazing.

Now imagine that as you're walking, you go to wherever it is that you're going to have your exercise session, whether it's the gym or the beach or for a bike ride or a walk or a swim, whatever it is you're going to be doing, and imagine that movement experience right now and how powerful you are and how energetic and how effortless it is. And you just can't stop running or walking or swimming or skipping or moving, and you have incredible strength and endurance and you can just see yourself in your most perfect, ideal shape glowing with energy. Your bones, your very bones are vibrating and glowing with energy you've got so much energy. And you know that you're going to have an incredible workout and the weight is just going to melt off your body now and you're going to finish your workout feeling calm, refreshed, energized, nourished, and effortlessly able to meet your weight loss goals and to have all the energy that you need to have an amazing day.

WEEK 9: REVERSE LEPTIN AND INSULIN RESISTANCE

NOTE—Use the Ocean of Energy visualization to get into SMART Mode. End this part of the visualization imagining every cell of your body glowing with white light . . .

And as your whole body is glowing with life force vitality, imagine now the actual cells of your body becoming more sensitive to the hormones leptin and insulin. Just imagine that on the outside of the cell walls there are little tiny receptors, like little tiny antennae that pop up all over the cell that make the cell very sensitive to the hormonal messages of these two hormones . . . First imagine it happening in one tiny cell, the antennae pop up all over the cell; just imagine that the same thing happens to all the other cells and this phenomenon spreads all over your body . . . 70 trillion cells all instantly becoming very sensitive to these crucial fat-regulating hormones . . .

You're using the power of your mind to reconfigure your cells, becoming like a naturally thin person, so you burn fat quickly and easily and you have effortless, boundless energy and you crave only the highest-quality, live, vibrant, nourishing foods.

As you imagine this sensitivity spreading to every cell, also imagine that the fat is now melting off your body. It's just dissolving into the earth and you're sitting there in your most perfect, ideal shape . . .

Imagine once again how every cell of your body now has more receptors, so the cells are very sensitive to the hormones leptin and insulin, and your body effortlessly burning fat and the weight, just melting off your body . . .

Now imagine yourself throughout the day, today and in the coming days and weeks, having lots of stable energy, craving only healthy, live, vibrant foods, and getting fitter, stronger, healthier, and more vibrant, day after day.

And in your own space and time, when you're ready, you can open your eyes.

WEEK 10: RELEASE TRAUMA

NOTE—Use the Ocean of Energy visualization to get into SMART Mode. End this part of the visualization imagining a ball of bright white light circulating around your navel and your body in an infinite ocean of energy . . .

And this light is so healing and protective and nurturing, and you feel safe being bathed in this beautiful white light. And you can imagine every cell of your body saying at the same time, "Safe, safe, safe, safe. I feel safe, safe, safe, safe. I feel safe. I feel safe." And you can imagine every cell of your body saying at the same time, "Love, love, love, love," like a concert or a chorus, 70 trillion cells all saying at the same time the words, "Love, love, love," and you can feel every cell of your body being bathed in love, and every cell of your body feeling safe and protected.

And as every cell of your body is feeling safe and protected, you can just imagine that every cell of your body lets go of any pain, any emotional trauma that's stored in the cells of your body; it just lets go and it gets washed away, in this beautiful ocean of bright white light. So you can imagine every cell of your body saying at the same time the words, "Let go, let go, let go. I let go, let go, let go. I release. I forgive. I forget. I move on."

So if you're willing, you can just allow every cell of your body to let go, to forgive, to move on. Forgiveness is really a gift that we give ourselves. Forgiveness is for us. Forgiveness is so we can move on. Forgiveness makes us lighter. Forgiveness makes life easier for us. Forgiveness is the ultimate healing tool that we have, to totally heal our body and to let go . . .

To let go of pain, to let go of trauma, and to let go of any additional weight that you're carrying on your body . . . So you can imagine every cell of your body letting go, and all that pain and trauma being washed away in this ocean of bright white light, never to be seen again. You've forgiven, you've let go, you've moved on, and you can see yourself getting thinner and thinner and thinner . . .

And so you can imagine yourself now losing weight and getting thinner and thinner and thinner. You can imagine all the excess weight just melting off your body. You don't need it anymore. You've let go. You've forgiven. You've moved on. You've released any emotional trauma out of the cells of your body, washed away never to be seen again. And you can see yourself walking on the street later today or maybe tomorrow, and you're happy, healthy, confident, fit, safe, secure, protected, nourished, vibrating with life force vitality, smiling . . . You're fit, happy, healthy. People can't help but notice how incredibly vibrant you are, and you can't help but notice how amazing you look and feel. You have so much energy, so much power, and the weight is just melting off your body.

And you can see over the next couple of days and weeks, how you're effortlessly becoming your ideal weight, now and always, and also all the while feeling safe and protected and nourished. You can feel how every cell of your body has released any emotional trauma, how every cell of your body is clean, happy, healthy, pure, vibrant, vibrating with life force vitality . . . And how you lose weight effortlessly, today and every day, until you have reached your ideal weight.

And so as you see yourself over the next couple of weeks getting fitter and fitter and fitter and thinner and happier and healthier, you know, beyond a shadow of a doubt, that you've released any pain that you needed to release . . . It's gone, never to be seen again—washed away in this ocean of light. And that ocean of light is bathing your cells, every minute of your day, giving you energy throughout the day and making you feel safe and protected, confident, happy, healthy, secure, and giving you vibrant health and vitality . . .

So in your own time and space, when you're ready, you can open your eyes, knowing that you've just totally transformed on a cellular level, that you've released any emotional trauma or pain that you've ever stored in your body. You've let go. You've moved on. You've cleansed yourself on a cellular level, and now weight loss will be effortless and automatic. And all you need to do is let it happen, and you let it happen easily and effortlessly.

And so in your own time and space, when you're ready, you can open your eyes, knowing that you've released any and all past issues that were holding you back, that on a cellular level, you've released and let go and your body has now transformed into a body that wants to be thin, fit, and vibrantly healthy and that loses weight easily and effortlessly and automatically.

WEEK 11: HEAL YOUR BODY

Just sitting up straight, I'd like you to imagine that there's a ball of bright white light in your navel, and it's just circulating around your navel and it's getting brighter and brighter and brighter. It looks like a galaxy of bright white light. And as this ball of bright white light is circulating around your navel, I'd like you to also imagine that you're in an infinite ocean of bright white light. That same bright white light that's in your navel is everywhere, as far as you can see, as far as you can imagine, in every direction is bright white healing light, ultrabright, and it's infinite.

And as you're sitting there, I'd just like you to imagine that the pores of your skin open up and all of this beautiful bright white light comes rushing into your body, filling your entire body with this beautiful, healing, luminescent energy . . . And this bright light is incredibly healing. So every cell of your body is being charged with this superbright white light. You can feel your bones and your arms being charged, and your bones and your hips and your legs starting to glow with bright white light. Your spine is glowing with bright light. Your ribs, your shoulders, your face, and all the bones in your head and your scalp are now glowing with superbright white light.

And your heart is getting charged with this light, and so your heart is glowing brighter and brighter, and all the blood that's rushing out of your heart into all the different parts of your body is supercharged with this bright white luminosity. So your blood is glowing with bright white light. And as it travels all through your body and it feeds your cells, your cells start to glow with this bright light. And everywhere this light touches it heals . . . so that any blockages that you have, any diseases, anything that's not functioning properly instantly vanishes as soon as this light touches it . . .

Like a bubble that's bursting. The second the light touches whatever is not good in your body, whatever needs to go away bursts like a bubble . . . So this white light travels down the left side of your body and the right side of your body and all through your body, and you're swimming in this ocean of bright light, and it's healing every cell of your body.

All of your energy channels that circulate through your body are unblocked and flowing . . . superhighways of energy going up and down your spine and through every little capillary of your body there's white light flowing. And it's touching every cell, and any cell that's not supposed to be there—pop—in an instant it vanishes, never to be seen again . . . Any bacteria that's not supposed to be there—pop—in an instant it vanishes. Any yeasts, parasites, mutated cells, all instantly vaporized, never to be seen again . . .

So all the blockages are cleared out, all the negative things are cleared out, any diseases are cleared out. They're all flushed out of your body, and you're sitting there in this ocean of white light and you can see your body is glowing with bright white light, totally healed, full of vitality, functioning perfectly well. Any toxins are instantly vaporized in this bright white light. Your body is renewed, regenerated, reenergized. In essence, you've got a new body, a body of light, and it feels so amazing . . .

And as you're sitting here totally charged, with superwhite, bright, healing life force light energy, as you're sitting here, I'd like you to imagine that any excess weight on your body just gets instantly vaporized into this ocean of white light. And you're sitting there in your most perfect, ideal shape . . . You don't need any excess weight anymore, because you've got energy. You're swimming in an ocean, an endless ocean of beautiful, bright energy. You don't need any excess weight anymore. You've got boundless energy.

Your energy channels are open. They're flowing all day long. You can imagine yourself all day long in your most perfect, ideal shape, having endless energy to be incredibly successful at work . . . to be productive and enjoy your family . . . to be out having fun with your friends, doing sports or just having fun, having a good time, traveling and just feeling happy, healthy, successful, and glowing with life force vitality . . .

And everyone you encounter feels this enormous energy that's coming out of you and they see how incredible you look, and people want to do business with you, they want to hang out with you, they want to enjoy your company, they just want to bask in your beautiful essence, glow that's coming out of you . . . They don't know what it is, but it's just radiating from you. You're a beautiful being of light now, totally clean, totally cleansed, pure . . . your body, mind, emotions, energy, all purified, and you're sitting there in your most perfect, ideal shape, just glowing with bright white light.

And as you're sitting there in your most perfect, ideal shape, just glowing with bright white life force energy, I'd like you to imagine that anytime during the day that you feel like you need energy you can tap into this ocean, so you never, ever run out of energy. And so you're no longer hungry for junk food. You don't need junk food to give you energy anymore, because you've tapped into the infinite source of energy that's all around you, and so you're getting fitter and fitter and happier and healthier and more vibrant, more relaxed, feeling safe, confident, and able to effortlessly have an incredibly successful, fit, happy, healthy, and productive life.

And in your own time and space, when you're ready, you can open your eyes, knowing that you forever transformed your body into a body of superlight life force energy, abundantly flowing, happy, infinitely healthy, peaceful, fit, successful, and content, now and forever.

WEEK 12: LOVE YOUR BODY

So if you're ready, just sitting up straight, take a deep breath in and a deep breath out and relax. I'd like you to imagine once again that there's a ball a beautiful white light circulating around your navel. And it's getting brighter and brighter and brighter. And as that ball of bright white light is circulating around your navel, I'd like you to imagine also that you're in an ocean of bright white light, as far as you can see, it's infinite in every direction, and it's bright white healing light. It might even be a slightly rose-colored light, which is the light of the color of love.

And this ocean is a loving, beautiful, nourishing ocean—a healing ocean. And as you're sitting there with this beautiful ball of bright white light in your navel and in this ocean of bright white and rose-colored light, I'd like you to imagine that the pores of your skin open up and this beautiful bright light, white and rose-colored light comes flooding into your body and fills your body with a beautiful, loving light.

You can feel every cell of your body being bathed with love. You can feel the bones in your feet being bathed with this loving light, and your knees and your thighs and the bones in your hips and your spine, as it runs up your spine into your shoulders and your arms. And your scalp and your face, your bones are just sucking it up, they're just being charged with a beautiful, loving, healing light.

And this light is flowing through your body, and everywhere this light touches your body is healed. Any blockages, any darkness, any negativity all gets washed away in the ocean of love. So that your muscles in your arms and your legs and in your torso and chest and your neck and in your face and your head, your muscles and tendons are being bathed with love, and your organs, you can feel your kidneys behind your stomach in your back, your kidneys are being bathed with love . . . Just take a moment to bathe your kidneys with love. They work so hard . . . And your adrenal glands right above your kidneys, they work so hard pumping out stress hormones all the time. Let's give them a moment of complete, utter love and bliss. Let's bathe our adrenal glands with love. Let them know that we're safe. They don't have to pump out stress hormones all the time; everything's okay now, just safety.

And feel that ocean of love going into your stomach and healing your stomach, clearing out any waste, unblocking any blockages, releasing any tension anywhere in your body. And your liver is being bathed with love, and your spleen and your lungs just being bathed with beautiful love, loving energy. It's an ocean of energy and it's going through you and around you and it's caressing every cell of your body. And your heart is being filled with this loving energy. And it's sending blood that's charged with a loving energy to every cell of your body.

And as this supercharged blood goes to every cell of your body, you can feel every cell of your body saying at the same time, "Love, love. I am love. I am forgiveness. I am acceptance. I am gratitude. I am appreciation. I am love. I am love, I am love." And feel every cell of your body say at the same time, "I am safe. I am safe. I am safe." . . .

So, every cell of your body, like a chorus, is saying at the same time, "I am love. I am safe. I am forgiveness. I am acceptance. I am appreciation. I am gratitude. I am love." And you can feel every cell of your body growing brighter and brighter. And healing, every cell of your body is being healed with love. And this love, like an ocean, is coursing through your body from all directions. And it's in your heart, and your heart, like a spotlight, is radiating light to every part of your body . . .

And as your body feels safe with love, you notice also that any excess weight on your body starts to melt off. It just dissolves in the ocean of love. And you're sitting there, in your most perfect, ideal shape . . . you're fit, you're strong, you're healthy, you're happy, you're confident. You're feeling tremendous love and support from the universe, from all directions. You're in an ocean of love and support. There's no way to escape it. Everywhere you turn, you're feeling love and support and protection and bliss and approval and appreciation. Everywhere you turn, it's an infinite ocean of love . . .

And as you're sitting there, totally bathed in love and every cell of your body radiating love, and as you're sitting there and all of your excess weight has been dissolved, I'd like you to imagine what your days are going to be like over the next couple of days, and over the next month as you're getting fitter and healthier. You can see yourself talking to someone and you're just radiating love, and they're mesmerized by the love that's coming out of you. And maybe you're at work, at a business meeting, and you're talking, and everyone is just spellbound by how beautiful you are and the beautiful energy that's coming out of you. And your family is loving toward you; they're reflecting the love back.

You've become a beacon of love. You've become a love generator. And everybody all around you is just basking in the glow of the beautiful love that you're emanating. And because your body feels so safe now, because it's being bathed in love, all the FAT programs are off, and the weight is just melting off your body. Your body wants to be thin and your body wants healthy foods, and you want to give your body the healthy foods that will love it even more, because it will nourish your body and make you feel even more loved . . .

And as the days go on and even the months, you're getting fitter and more and more successful and happy and healthy and vibrant and peaceful and radiating energy, vitality, beauty, and love. This love is an ocean, and you feel it everywhere. And anytime you need to feel it, you just open up your pores and allow it to come in. It's always there for you and you always feel it, and from now on you feel loved and supported and protected and nourished, now and forever. And your life is getting better and better and better . . . And you can see it from day to day, you're getting fitter and healthier and more successful and happier and more in control. And in every possible way you're improving.

So in your own time and space, when you're ready, you can open your eyes, knowing that you're forever bathed in an ocean of love . . . And that your body is radiating this love out into the world . . . And that this love is guiding you toward success, happiness, fitness, health, and vitality. So when you're ready, please open your eyes and know that you have connected with a source of love that is forever there for you, and that you're going to have a tremendous month of fitness, health, and vitality.

WEEK 13: ELIMINATE CRAVINGS AND ADDICTIONS

CAUTION—This visualization uses unpleasant imagery to create a negative association with foods and substances you'd like to avoid. Please only listen to this visualization if you feel it's appropriate for you.

NOTE—Use the Ocean of Energy visualization to get into SMART Mode. End this part of the visualization imagining a ball of bright white light circulating around your navel and your body in an infinite ocean of energy . . .

And as you're sitting there, with this ball of light in your navel, and it's spinning around, like a whirlpool or a galaxy, I'd like you to imagine that any excess weight you have on your body is being sucked into this ball of light, never to be seen again. It's pulling excess weight you have, in your legs, your arms, your back, your chest, your stomach, all getting sucked into this whirlpool, never to be seen again.

And you're sitting there, in your most perfect, ideal shape . . . And as you're sitting there in your most perfect, ideal shape, I'd like you to imagine that you're going for a walk during the day. It could be a typical day. You're walking down the street, you're talking to your friends, and you're feeling fit, healthy, vibrant, and happy . . . And you come across a store that has the type of food that you'd like to avoid. It could be a bakery or a fast-food restaurant, or just a convenience store, whatever it is. You see yourself walking into that store, and getting whatever the food is, and you open it up, and you take a bite of it . . . and the second you touch it to your tongue, you realize there's something wrong with it. It tastes repulsive. You look at the food and you notice something is very wrong . . . Maybe there are some bugs or worms in the food or it's moldy, or if it's chocolate, you realize it's actually dirt . . .

. . . Just take a moment to see the scene in as graphic detail as possible. Use your imagination and come up with a scenario that's as repulsive as you can imagine . . . Then imagine instantly spitting the food out of your mouth and being disgusted by it . . . You can try this with a few different foods if you like . . . Just imagine that now if you want [30 second pause].

You can also imagine this with other substances, like smoking or drinking. Just take a moment now to do that if appropriate . . .

Now imagine that same scene on another day . . . You're walking down the street and you're feeling fit, happy, healthy, protected, nurtured, supported, loved, bursting with energy and life and vitality and you walk by the same store and you notice the food that you used to be attracted to and the second you look at it, you feel disgusted . . . Maybe your stomach knots up; you don't want to be anywhere near it . . . You feel repulsed by that food or substance now. You can't even walk near the store. You don't want any part of that, and you walk past . . .

. . . And instead you see yourself craving healthy, live, vibrant, beautiful foods . . . foods that will sustain you, foods that will nourish you, and you feel your body being nourished and sustained by these foods—real, live, healthy, vibrant foods are what your body is now craving, and you can see yourself being sustained and nourished and supported by these foods, and energized all through the day . . .

And all the weight is just melting off you effortlessly. You love the food that you're eating now—healthy, live, vibrant foods. You're drinking lots of water, and you feel incredible. And you see how, day by day, you're getting healthier, and fitter, and happier, and more vibrant. And the weight's just melting off your body, day by day. And as each day goes by, you crave healthier foods, more live foods. The more vibrant you become, the healthier the foods you like; you can see yourself day after day, getting fitter, healthier, more energy, more alive, and more vibrant . . . You're bursting with life, you're bursting with vitality, you're exploding with love for life and into the world, and everything in your life is flowing, now and always.

And in your own time and space, when you're ready, you can open your eyes knowing that you just totally just transformed your body on a cellular level to crave healthy, live, vibrant foods, real foods. And so you're feeling enormous energy and life force vitality in your body, and the weight is now effortlessly melting off your body. And any food that once gave you trouble is the furthest thing from your mind right now. In fact, it's repulsive. You don't want to be anywhere near it. And you just gravitate more and more toward healthy, live, beautiful, vibrant, fresh foods. And your body is transforming at every level.

And in your own time and space, you can open your eyes, and have a beautiful day.

WEEK 14: CREATE VIBRANT, ELASTIC SKIN

NOTE—Use the Ocean of Energy visualization to get into SMART Mode. End this part of the visualization imagining a ball of bright white light circulating around your navel and your body in an infinite ocean of energy . . .

And as you're sitting there, with your entire body just glowing with this beautiful bright white healing light, and with this ball of bright white light circulating around your navel like a vortex or a whirlpool of energy, I'd like you to imagine that any excess weight you have on your body just gets sucked into this whirlpool of energy. It's like a black hole that sucks any excess weight into your body so you can feel any excess weight that you have on your legs getting sucked into this whirlpool or this vortex. You can feel any excess weight you have on your pelvis or your stomach just getting sucked into this vortex. And you can feel any excess weight you have on your chest or your arms, or your face; it's all just becoming like a liquid light. It's almost like a bright white light energy, and it's just getting sucked into the vortex in your navel, never to be seen again. And you're sitting there in your most perfect, ideal shape . . .

And as you're sitting there, in your most perfect, ideal shape, in this ocean of energy, and with any excess weight just being sucked into the vortex in your navel, I'd like you to also imagine any excess skin you have on your body becomes like a rose-colored light that also gets sucked into this vortex in your navel; so this excess skin gets sucked in, gets pulled into this vortex. And your skin is tight and toned . . . So you can feel this vortex just pulling any excess loose skin from your stomach or your pelvis or your arms or your legs or your chest or your face, just pulling it into your navel. And you can feel, and you can imagine that your stomach is tight as a drum; there's no excess skin. You can't even pinch any excess skin on your wrist. There's no excess skin. It's just tight and toned . . .

And as you're sitting there, in your most perfect, ideal shape, with your skin toned and tight, I'd like you to imagine, in your mind's eye, that you go for a walk on the beach. And you can see and feel how your body is firm and toned . . . You can see your skin as tight against your body, super, super tight. And you can see yourself in your most perfect, ideal shape. And you're just going for a walk on the beach, and just feeling what it feels like to have your most perfect, ideal body and your most perfect, ideal shape.

And you can imagine your day tomorrow, or later today, going beautifully and you in your most perfect, ideal shape. You can imagine your skin getting tighter and more toned and the weight just melting off your body, and you're craving only healthy, live, vibrant foods . . . And you're feeling super alive and vibrant and having an amazing day, whether you're at work in business, or with your family and friends, everything flowing beautifully; lots of energy, or excitement, or vitality, and the weight just melting off your body . . .

And you can imagine the coming days, the coming weeks, and this weight just melting off your body day by day, and your skin is getting toned and tight and firm. And how you have this vortex in your navel all the time, always pulling your skin in tighter and more toned. Your skin is alive, vibrant, superhealthy, superelastic. It's growing with beautiful life force vitality. Your whole body is glowing with life force vitality . . . Your bones are glowing, your muscles and your ligaments and your organs and your skin, all glowing with a beautiful, live, vibrant life force vitality. And you can even just imagine, day after day, and week after week, how you're getting fitter, healthy, stronger, and your skin is getting more toned and more tight, until you easily and naturally reach your ideal body . . .

And in your own time and space, when you're ready, you can open your eyes, knowing that you've just used the power of your mind to create a body that's toned and tight and firm . . . That your skin will now become tighter and more elastic and more vibrant; that you've got this vortex in your navel that's always pulling excess weight into it and always pulling your skin tighter and tighter, and that you will lose weight, easily and naturally . . . And your skin will get tighter and more elastic easily, and you'll get fitter effortlessly and easily, day after day, until you have reached your most perfect, ideal body.

WEEK 15: INSPIRE ABUNDANCE

NOTE—Use the Ocean of Energy visualization to get into SMART Mode. End this part of the visualization imagining a ball of bright white light circulating around your navel and your body in an infinite ocean of energy . . .

Now imagine that this ocean of energy you are in is actually an ocean of infinite abundance. And anything you'd like to achieve, whether it's more financial freedom, more loving relationships, more success in business or in personal life, or more health and vitality and happiness, this ocean of abundance instantly transforms into the very thing you would like to achieve.

So if it's financial freedom you want, imagine you're in an ocean of prosperity, and just one drop of that ocean is more financial freedom, more success financially than you could ever imagine or ever need in an entire life, just one drop . . . If it's a more loving relationship you want, imagine one drop is more love than you could ever possibly need or want in your entire life . . . If it's success in business, one drop is more success than you ever imagined possible; just one drop and you're in an infinite ocean of success, abundance, happiness, wealth, prosperity, and fitness . . .

And I'd like you to imagine that you open the pores of your skin and all that prosperity, success, wealth, happiness, and fitness comes rushing into you. All you need to do is allow it in. It's everywhere. It's an ocean of success and fitness. It's infinite and it's everywhere, and all you need to do is allow that to come in . . . And you open up the pores of your skin and you allow that energy to come through you, and it comes through you and it rushes into your life, creating success in every aspect of your life—financial success, success in business, success in relationships, fitness, family life, health, and vitality, success in every aspect of your life . . .

This ocean floods through you, energizing and empowering every aspect of your life. And now you're using the power of your mind to create everything you want in your life, and now all you have to do is let it in . . .

So imagine now, this ocean of abundance rushing into your body and out into the world, creating success in every way possible . . . And now imagine yourself and your life in six months from now . . . See how you've lost all your excess weight, and you're successful in every aspect of your life . . . Professionally you're doing exactly what you would like to be doing. Your relationships and your family life are harmonious. Your friendships are fun and joyful. If there are any career changes you'd like to make, if there are any career goals that you have, imagine all of them have been achieved times 10 million . . . So much more than you ever thought possible, and you can't even imagine how successful you are . . . And you've got happiness and energy and vitality and people are coming up to you and they're listening to you and they're respecting you and they're getting the information you're giving them and it's helping them, and you're directing them and you're in charge of the life you want to be in charge of and you're amazingly successful . . . You're doing the business you want to do with them, and there's love between you and your family members and your relationships . . .

And as you're looking at this picture that you've just created of this ideal life, that's being energized by this ocean of abundance that you're in, imagine that this scene of your ideal life is like a magnet that's drawing you, so that every decision you make from now on, whether you turn left or whether you turn right, whether you talk to this person or go on this vacation or go to this restaurant . . . every single decision you make you're making because that magnet is pulling you to your most ideal, successful, happy, fit, prosperous, enjoyable, energetic, healthy, and happy life.

And in your own time and space, you can open your eyes knowing that forever, for the rest of your life, you will be bathing in this infinite ocean of abundance and you will be tremendously successful in every aspect of your life.

WEEK 16: BECOME YOUR FULL POTENTIAL

NOTE—Use the Ocean of Energy visualization to get into SMART Mode. End this part of the visualization imagining a ball of bright white light circulating around your navel and your body in an infinite ocean of energy . . .

And you can imagine every cell of your body saying at the same time the words, "Success, success, success. I am success, success, success. I allow, I allow, I allow." And you can imagine every cell of your body saying at the same time, "I allow greatness into my life. I allow myself to be great. I allow greatness. I allow every cell of my body to become great." . . .

And you can imagine how this greatness is manifesting. And you can see yourself in the coming days being enormously successful in whatever it is that you're passionate about . . . You're living up to your true potential, in every aspect of the word, and you can see how day after day you're becoming healthier, happier, and more successful.

And you can see yourself being successful and losing weight. How day after day, the weight is just melting off your body, and professionally how your career is growing in enormous ways. How you're giving and learning and sharing and following your true purpose. You can see how your purpose is being manifested in the world, and you just allow it to come through . . . And it's almost as if this ocean of energy that's coming through your body is guiding you and coming through you, to manifest greatness and to help you be and become your full potential, in every aspect of life.

So you can see yourself, day after day in the coming days and months, getting fitter and healthier . . . And you can see how you're truly living up to your potential. In fitness—becoming superfit, superhealthy, superhappy. You can see yourself living up to and becoming your full potential in your relationships with your loved ones—as a parent if you're a parent, as a lover, as a friend, as a member of your community . . .

Professionally, your life is expanding in ways that you never thought possible . . . growing and expanding. You're on a mission. You see this energy coming through you, and you can see yourself maybe in six months from now, being fit, healthy, happy, and living your full potential . . . You can see the energy, this ocean of energy, coming through you, and you're just exploding with life force and love and passion for everything it is that you want to be and do and give to the world . . . You're just exploding with light and love, and everyone you touch, everyone you see, feels it, and they're bathed in this life and they're transformed . . .

And you can see yourself just spreading this enormous light and beauty and power throughout the world . . . This is your full potential. It's coming through you like an explosion of energy, manifesting in so many incredible ways, in creativity . . . in productivity . . . in health . . . in happiness . . . in guidance . . . in transformation . . .

. . . Transformation for yourself and transformation for the world. You've become a light for the world, a beacon for the world.

You are a beacon of light for this world and this universe, and this beautiful light comes through you and it transforms everything, from trees to people to birds, entire countries are being transformed because this light is coming through you and you are living up to your full potential in every conceivable way.

So in your own time and space, when you're ready, you can open your eyes, knowing that you've just connected with this infinite ocean of energy, and this infinite ocean of energy is coming through you and exploding through you, to help you become your full potential, in every aspect of the word . . . To become fitter, healthier, happier, smarter, more loving, more giving . . . To be exploding with passion in every aspect of your life, and to be a light for yourself, your family, your loved ones, and the world. And to be your full potential in every sense of the word, now and always . . .

NOTES

Chapter 1: Lose Weight from the Inside-Out

1. Zheng, H., "Appetite Control and Energy Balance Regulation in the Modern World: Reward-Driven Brain Overrides Repletion Signals," *International Journal of Obesity* 33, suppl. 2 (June 2009): S8–13.

2. Ibid.

3. Ibid.

4. Ibid.

Chapter 2: Why Visualization Works

1. Arnold Schwarzenegger, *The New Encyclopedia of Modern Bodybuilding* (New York: Simon & Schuster, 1998): 402.

Chapter 3: Melt Stress, Melt Fat

1. Sleye, H., "A Syndrome Produced by Diverse Noxious Agents," *Nature* 138 (1936): 32.

2. Shively C.A., et al., "Social Stress, Visceral Obesity, and Coronary Artery Atherosclerosis in Female Primates," *Obesity* 17, no. 8 (August 2009): 1513–1520.

3. Block, J.P., et al., "Psychosocial Stress and Change in Weight Among US Adults," *American Journal of Epidemiology* 170 (2009): 181–192.

4. Tomiyama, A.J., et al., "Comfort Food Is Comforting to Those Most Stressed: Evidence of the Chronic Stress Response Network in High-Stress Women," *Psychoneuroendocrinology* 36, no. 10 (November 2011): 1513–1519.

5. Pankevich, D.E., et al., "Caloric Restriction Experience Reprograms Stress and Orexegenic Pathways and Promotes Binge-Eating," *Journal of Neuroscience* 30, no. 48 (December 1, 2010): 16,399–16,407.

6. Nyklíček, I., et al., "Mindfulness-based Stress Reduction and Physiological Activity During Acute Stress: A Randomized Controlled Trial," *Health Psychology* 32, no. 10 (October 2013): 1110–1113.

7. Foureur, M., et al., "Enhancing the Resilience of Nurses and Midwives: Pilot of Mindfulness-Based Program for Increased Health, Sense of Coherence and Decreased Depression, Anxiety and Stress," *Contemporary Nurse* 45, no. 1 (August 2013): 114–125.

8. Hölzel, B.K., et al., "Neural Mechanisms of Symptom Improvements in Generalized Anxiety Disorder Following Mindfulness Training," *NeuroImage: Clinical* 2 (2013): 448–458.

9. Rosenkranz, M.A., et al., "A Comparison of Mindfulness-Based Stress Reduction and an Active Control in Modulation of Neurogenic Inflammation," *Brain, Behavior, and Immunity* 27 (2013): 174–184.

10. Daubenmier, J., et al., "Mindfulness Intervention for Stress Eating to Reduce Cortisol and Abdominal Fat among Overweight and Obese Women: An Exploratory Randomized Controlled Study," *Journal of Obesity* 2011 (2011): doi:10.1155/2011/651936.

Chapter 4: Overcome Trauma and Fear

1. Lumeng, J.C., et al., "Overweight Adolescents and Life Events in Childhood," *Pediatrics* (November 11, 2013): doi: 10.1542/peds.2013-1111.

2. Williamson, D.F., et al., "Body Weight and Obesity in Adults and Self-reported Abuse in Childhood," *International Journal of Obesity and Related Metabolic Disorders* 26, no. 8 (August 2002): 1075–1082.

3. Hund, A.R., Espelage, D.L., "Childhood Emotional Abuse and Disordered Eating Among Undergraduate Females: Mediating Influence of Alexithymia and Distress," *Child Abuse and Neglect* 30, no 4. (April 2006): 393–407.

4. Flitti V.J., et al., "Childhood Sexual Abuse, Depression, and Family Dysfunction in Adult Obese Patients: A Case Control Study," *Southern Medical Journal* 86, no. 7 (July 1993): 732–736.

Chapter 5: Tap into the Biology of Your Beliefs

1. Milton, G.W., "Self-Willed Death or the Bone-Pointing Syndrome," *Lancet* 1, no. 7817 (June 23, 1973): 1435–1436.

2. Reeves, R.R. et al., "Nocebo Effects with Antidepressant Drugs," *General Hospital Psychiatry* 29, no. 3 (May–June 2007): 2757.

3. Story related by Wayne Dyer in Hay House Radio interview.

4. *The Living Matrix—The Science of Healing*, dir. Greg Becker, Emaginate, 2010.

5. Sarris, J., et al., "St. John's Wort Versus Sertraline and Placebo in Major Depressive Disorder: Continuation Data From a 26-Week RCT," *Pharmacopsychiatry* 45, no. 7 (November 2012): 275–280.

6. Kirsch, I., et al., "Initial Severity and Antidepressant Benefits: A Meta-Analysis of Data Submitted to the Food and Drug Administration," *PLOS Medicine* 5, no. 2 (February 26, 2008): 0260–0267.

7. Lidstone, S.C., "Effects of Expectation on Placebo-Induced Dopamine Release in Parkinson Disease," *Archives of General Psychiatry* 67, no. 8 (August 2010): 857–865.

8. Dawson Church, *The Genie in Your Genes* (Santa Rosa, CA: Energy Psychology Press, 2009): 126.

9. *The Living Matrix.*

10. Crum, J.A., and E.J. Langer, "Mind-Set Matters: Exercise and the Placebo Effect," *Psychological Science* 18, no. 2 (2007): 165–171.

Chapter 7: Pathways to Healthy Habits

1. Bruce E. Wexler, *Brain and Culture: Neurobiology, Ideology, and Social Change*, (Cambridge, MA: MIT Press, 2006).

2. Spring, B., et al., "Multiple Behavior Change in Diet and Activity: A Randomized Controlled Trial Using Mobile Technology," *Archives of Internal Medicine* 172, no. 10 (May 28, 2012): 789–796.

3. Ornish, D., et al., "Effect of Comprehensive Lifestyle Changes on Telomerase Activity and Telomere Length in Men with Biopsy-Proven Low-Risk Prostate Cancer: 5-Year Follow-Up of a Descriptive Pilot Study," *The Lancet Oncology* 14, no. 11 (October 2013): 1112–1120.

4. Schwabe, L., et al., "Simultaneous Glucocorticoid and Noradrenergic Activity Disrupts the Neural Basis of Goal-Directed Action in the Human Brain," *Journal of Neuroscience* 32, no. 30 (July 25, 2012): 10,146–10,155.

Chapter 8: Rediscover the Joy of Movement

1. Emily Benammar, "Didier Drogba Missing Chances for Chelsea Because of Concentration Lapses," *The Telegraph* online (October 14, 2008): www .telegraph.co.uk/sport/football/teams/chelsea/3193860/Didier-Drogba -missing-chances-for-Chelsea-because-of-concentration-lapses-Football. html.

2. Yao, W.X., et al., "Kinesthetic Imagery Training of Forceful Muscle Contractions Increases Brain Signal and Muscle Strength," *Frontiers in Human Neuroscience* 7, no. 561 (September 2013): doi: 10.3389/fnhum.

3. Ranganathan V.K. et al., "From Mental Power to Muscle Power: Gaining Strength by Using the Mind," *Neuropsychologia* 42, no. 7 (2004): 944–956.

4. U.S. Department of Health and Human Services, National Institutes of Health, National Heart, Lung, and Blood Institute, "Aim for a Healthy Weight: Key Recommendations," (1998): www.nhlbi.nih.gov/health/public/heart/obesity/lose_wt/recommen.htm.

5. Little, J.P., et al., "A Practical Model of Low-Volume High-Intensity Interval Training Induces Mitochondrial Biogenesis in Human Skeletal Muscle: Potential Mechanisms," *Journal of Physiology* 588, no. 6 (March 2010): 1011–1022.

6. Ibid.

7. Cocks, M., et al., "Sprint Interval and Endurance Training Are Equally Effective in Increasing Muscle Microvascular Density and eNOS Content in Sedentary Males," *Journal of Physiology* 591, no. 3 (February 1, 2013): 641–656.

8. Trapp E.G., et al., "The Effects of High-Intensity Intermittent Exercise Training on Fat Loss and Fasting Insulin Levels of Young Women," *International Journal of Obesity* 32, no. 4 (2008): 684–691.

Chapter 9: Sleep Your Way to Slenderness

1. Brown, M.A., et al., "The Impact of Sleep-Disordered Breathing on Body Mass Index: The Sleep Heart Health Study," *Southwest Journal of Pulmonary and Critical Care* 3 (December 8, 2011): 159–168.

2. Taheri, S., et al., "Short Sleep Duration Is Associated with Reduced Leptin, Elevated Ghrelin, and Increased Body Mass Index," *PLOS Medicine* 1, no. 3 (December 2004): 210–217.

3. Spiegel, K., et al., "Brief Communication: Sleep Curtailment in Healthy Young Men Is Associated with Decreased Leptin Levels, Elevated Ghrelin Levels, and Increased Hunger and Appetite," *Annals of Internal Medicine* 141 (December 7, 2004): 846–850.

4. Nedeltcheva, A.V., et al., "Insufficient Sleep Undermines Dietary Efforts to Reduce Adiposity," *Annals of Internal Medicine* 153 (October 5, 2010): 435–441.

5. Weiss, A., et al., "The Association of Sleep Duration with Adolescents' Fat and Carbohydrate Consumption," *Sleep* 33, no. 9 (2010): 1201–1209.

6. Ayas, N.T., et al., "A Prospective Study of Sleep Duration and Coronary Heart Disease in Women," *Archives of Internal Medicine* 163, no. 2 (January 27, 2003): 205–209.

7. Watanabe, M., et al., "Association of Short Sleep Duration with Weight Gain and Obesity at 1-Year Follow-Up: A Large-Scale Prospective Study," *Sleep* 33, no. 2 (2010): 161–167.

8. Weiss, "The Association of Sleep . . . "

9. Gourineni, R., et al., "Effects of Meditation on Sleep in Individuals with Chronic Insomnia," presented at *SLEEP 2009*, the 23rd Annual Meeting of the Associated Professional Sleep Societies, Abstract ID: 0874.

10. Gross, C.R., et al., "Mindfulness-Based Stress Reduction vs. Pharmacotherapy for Primary Chronic Insomnia: A Pilot Randomized Controlled Clinical Trial," *Explore (NY)* 7, no. 2 (2011): 76–87.

11. Ibid.

Chapter 10: Overcome Food Cravings and Addictions

1. Harvey, K., et al., "The Nature of Imagery Processes Underlying Food Cravings," *British Journal of Health Psychology* 10, pt. 1 (February 2005): 49–56.

2. McClelland A., et al., "Reduction of Vividness and Associated Craving in Personalized Food Imagery," *Journal of Clinical Psychology* 62, no. 3 (March 2006): 355–365.

3. Pelchat, M.L., et al., "Images of Desire: Food-Craving Activation During fMRI," *Neuroimage* 23, no. 4 (December 2004): 1486–1493.

4. Sullum, Jacob, "Research Shows Cocaine and Heroin Are Less Addictive Than Oreos," *Forbes* (October 16, 2013): www.forbes.com/sites/jacobsullum/2013/10/16/research-shows-cocaine-and-heroin-are-less-addictive-than-oreos.

5. Kominars, K.D., "A Study of Visualization and Addiction Treatment," *Journal of Substance Abuse Treatment* 14, no. 3 (May–June 1997): 213–223.

Chapter 12: The Greater World of Mind-Body Practices

1. Ornish, D.M., et al., "Can Lifestyle Changes Reverse Coronary Atherosclerosis? The Lifestyle Heart Trial," *The Lancet* 336 (1990): 129–133.

2. Tran, M.D., et al., "Effects of Hatha Yoga Practice on the Health-Related Aspects of Physical Fitness," *Preventive Cardiology* 4, no. 4 (Autumn 2001): 165–170.

3. Kristal, A., et al., "Yoga Practice Is Associated with Attenuated Weight Gain in Healthy, Middle-Aged Men and Women," *Alternative Therapies in Health and Medicine* 11, no. 4 (July–August 2005): 28–33.

4. Framson, C., et al., "Development and Validation of the Mindful Eating Questionnaire," *Journal of the American Dietetic Association* 109, no. 8 (2009): 1439.

5. Edelman, D., et al., "Innovative Models of Health Care Study: A Multifaceted Intervention to Reduce Cardiovascular Risks in High Risk Individuals," *Journal of General Internal Medicine* 21 (July 2006): 728–734.

6. Desbordes, G., et al., "Effects of Mindful-Attention and Compassion Meditation Training on Amygdala Response to Emotional Stimuli in an Ordinary, Non-Meditative State," *Frontiers in Human Neuroscience* 6, art. 292 (November 1, 2012): doi: 10.3389/fnhum.2012.00292.

7. Kozhevnikov, M., et al., "The Enhancement of Visuospatial Processing Efficiency Through Buddhist Deity Meditation," *Psychological Science* 20, no. 5 (2009): 645–653.

8. Dawson Church, *The Genie in Your Genes*, 126–127.

Chapter 13: Intuitive Weight Loss

1. Office of Naval Research Basic Research Challenge—Enhancing Intuitive Decision Making Through Implicit Learning; Solicitation No. 12-SN-0007 (July 31, 2012): www.fbo.gov/index?s=opportunity&mode=form&tab=core &id=723de7fc46213a209552d9131dcf2132&_cview=0.

2. PRWeek: CEO Survey 2006, Burson-Marsteller: media.haymarketmedia. com/archives/1/2006ceosurvey_305.pdf.

3. McCraty, R., et. al., "Electrophysiological Evidence of Intuition: Part 1. The Surprising Role of the Heart," *Journal of Alternative and Complementary Medicine* 10, no. 1 (February 2004): 133–143.

ACKNOWLEDGMENTS

So many beautiful people contributed to the creation of this book and I'd just like to name a few of them here:

First and foremost, I'd like to thank my editors: John Hastings, Laura Gray, and Sherri Kronfeld; the design and publishing team at Hay House; my co-workers, support staff, and coaching team, especially Lucas Rockwood, Denaleigh Beard, Aeron McFarlene, Shannon Hawkes, Geraldine Navarrette, Janine Oliver, Brian Killian, Christine Kennedy, Smita Patel, Marjolijn Loderichs, Desiree Manders, Heather Flemming, Nadia Harper, Paula Robbins, Jennifer Welch, and Melinda Jacobs; my meditation and visualization teachers and inspirations, including Rafael Nasser, Robert Peng, Phoc Phan, Mantak Chia, Michael Winn, Hariharananda, Prajnananda, Don Abrams, John Williams, Tony Robbins, Arnold Schwarzenegger, Ramakrishna, Sarada Devi, Ananda Moy Ma, Guru Mai, Sri Chinmoy, Vivekananda, Yogananda, and Sri Yukteswar.

I'd also like to thank Inge Tatiana Abrams; Leonard, Ethel, Jennifer, Joe, and Michelle Abrams; Sharon Humpheys; Daphne Motskin; Jonathan Dichter; Kate Reardon; James Colquhoun; Laurentine Colquhoun Ten Bosch; Prince Hugo Maris Gabriel Colquhoun; Michael and Ellysia Maddens; Khaliah Ali; Uzi Silber; Eli Catalan; Gadi and Lalita Barak; Dr. Mark Hyman; Jason Vale; Dr. Christiane Northrup; Brittany Watkins; Dr. Sara Gottfried; JJ Virgin; Louise Hay; Reid Tracy; Kris Carr; Dr. Joseph Mercola; Dr. Ron Rosedale; Dr. Dawson Church; Dr. Howard Leibowitz; and the Institute of HeartMath.

I am extremely grateful for your contributions to this book, my work, and my life. Without your help, this book would not have been possible.

Last but most definitely not least I'd like to thank the thousands (if not millions at this point) of people who listen to and practice my visualizations on a daily basis. You continue to inspire me in ways you cannot possibly imagine!

ABOUT THE AUTHOR

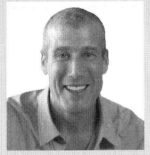

Jon Gabriel has a bachelor of science in economics from the Wharton School of the University of Pennsylvania. While there, he also pursued extensive coursework in biochemistry and performed research for the internationally recognized biochemist Dr Jose Rabinowitz.

In 1990 Jon started gaining weight for no apparent reason. He tried every diet and programme he could to lose weight, but in the end, he just kept gaining. The more he dieted, the more he gained.

The situation became critical in mid-2001 when he became morbidly obese and reached a weight of more than 400 pounds. On September 11, 2001, he was scheduled to fly from Newark to San Francisco, and it was only by a fluke of fate that he was not on United Airlines Flight 93, which was hijacked by terrorists.

This event, as well as some equally life-changing events that occurred in the weeks following 9/11, affected him deeply. It was this wake-up call that made him realize life was a precious opportunity not to be wasted. He decided to start 'living the life of his dreams'. He also decided to apply all his research skills and scientific background toward understanding and eliminating the real reasons he was fat.

The result is arguably one of the most remarkable physical transformations of all time. Jon lost more than 220 pounds without restrictive dieting and without surgery. Amazingly, his body shows almost no signs of ever being overweight at all – a fact that has astounded many professionals in the medical community.

Using the approach that has worked so well for him, he has now made it his life's mission to assist others in achieving tremendous success, not only in weight loss but in every aspect of life.

What started out as Jon's own weight loss story has now become an international movement for holistic, sustainable health and weight loss. Jon's first book, *The Gabriel Method*, is an international bestseller that's been translated into 16 languages and is sold in 60 countries.

www.thegabrielmethod.com

DO YOU HAVE QUESTIONS ABOUT THIS BOOK?

Talk Directly to Jon Gabriel in his Support Group

Have you ever heard the expression, "You become the sum of your three closest friends?" When it comes to your health, this couldn't be more true.

With this challenge in mind, many Gabriel Method readers find it essential to join a group of like-minded people to support them in their weight-loss journey. To help with this process, Jon Gabriel created a private, on-line Support Group back in 2011, and to date, it's been a tremendous help to thousands.

Over the years, the Support Group has grown into the central hub for all things Gabriel Method. This online community has members from 28 countries with expert classes, recipes, new visualizations, forum discussions, and regular opportunities each month to write in or call Jon himself.

This is Jon's virtual home for all his latest research, and it contains the most comprehensive library of Gabriel Method resources anywhere.

To learn more about The Gabriel Method Support Group and how you can get a FREE 30-day trial, visit: www.TheGabrielMethod.com/free-support-group-trial

READER BONUS:

THE "NEW YOU" VIDEO SERIES

FREE Online Video Classes with Jon Gabriel

Get instant access to this four-part webinar series produced by Jon Gabriel. Originally, these video classes were created for Jon's private coaching clients, but they give such a well-rounded overview of the core Gabriel Method principles that Jon decided to make them freely available to all his readers worldwide. The Video Class Topics Include:

- How to Release Weight 1lb at a Time
- Heal the Past, Lose the Weight
- The "Have it All" (un)Diet Secret to Eating
- No More Cardio (Gabriel Method Fitness 101)

To access from your phone or computer, please visit:
www.TheGabrielMethod.com/new-you

Other Hay House Titles to Inspire You

SLIMMING MEALS THAT HEAL: Lose Weight Without Dieting, Using Anti-inflammatory Superfoods by Julie Daniluk RHN

Diets fail because they are a self-imposed temporary food prison that people can't wait to escape. *Slimming Meals That Heal* will shatter the need to count calories and will conquer cravings. Nutritionist Julie Daniluk's clients who have followed the SMTH anti-inflammatory plan have lost 25, 45 and even 100 pounds.

Slimming Meals That Heal deepens readers' understanding of how food can hurt or heal. The book includes information on cleansing the organs, the power of superfoods and techniques that directly reduce cravings. Julie has devised a 5-step plan for how to boost metabolism and regulate hormones that leads to holistic weight balance.

—

THE TAPPING SOLUTION FOR WEIGHT LOSS AND BODY CONFIDENCE: A Woman's Guide to Stressing Less, Weighing Less and Loving More by Jessica Ortner

Jessica Ortner, producer of the highly successful documentary on meridian tapping, *The Tapping Solution*, offers women a better choice. Why not lose the weight and create the life you've always dreamt of? In this groundbreaking book, Jessica uses tapping to help tackle the stress that leads to weight gain – including the personal stresses of low self-esteem and a lack of confidence. Using her own struggles with weight loss, along with success stories of some of the thousands of women she's worked with, Jessica walks readers through the process of discovering their personal power and self-worth. Her programme is based on extensive research into the benefits and success of tapping and the hormones involved in stress and weight gain and it covers everything from the emotional aspects of overeating and cravings, to how to find joy in exercise, the power of pleasure and how our families and friends may inadvertently add to the problem.

Join the
HAY HOUSE
Family

As the leading self-help, mind, body and spirit publisher in the UK, we'd like to welcome you to our community so that you can keep updated with the latest news, including new releases, exclusive offers, author events and more.

Sign up at www.hayhouse.co.uk/register

Like us on Facebook at Hay House UK

Follow us on Twitter @HayHouseUK

www.hayhouse.co.uk

Hay House Publishers
Astley House, 33 Notting Hill Gate, London W11 3JQ
020 3675 2450   info@hayhouse.co.uk

Printed in Great Britain
by Amazon

51267514R00129